I AM A WOMAN
Creative, Sacred & Invincible

Kundalini Yoga as taught by *Yogi Bhajan*®

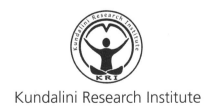

Kundalini Research Institute

ESSENTIAL KRIYAS **FOR WOMEN IN THE AQUARIAN AGE**

I AM A WOMAN: CREATIVE, SACRED, INVINCIBLE
ESSENTIAL KRIYAS FOR WOMEN IN THE AQUARIAN AGE

FIRST EDITION Copyright © 2009 Kundalini Research Institute

EDITOR
Sat Purkh Kaur Khalsa
Kundalini Research Institute

SENIOR EDITORIAL BOARD
Pritpal Kaur Khalsa, Guru Raj Kaur Khalsa, Dev Suroop Kaur Khalsa, Deva Kaur Khalsa,
Hari Charn Kaur Khalsa & Tarn Taran Kaur Khalsa

CONSULTING EDITORS & CONTRIBUTORS
Ek Ong Kaar Kaur Khalsa, Siri Neel Kaur Khalsa (KRI Review), Shakti Parwha Kaur Khalsa, Gurucharan Kaur Khalsa,
Gurucharan Singh Khalsa, Harbhajan Kaur Khalsa (Millis), Nam Nidhan Kaur Khalsa (Chile), Nirvair Singh Khalsa

COPY EDITOR
Guru Raj Kaur Khalsa

GURMUKHI EDITORS
Guru Raj Kaur Khalsa & Guru Sangat Kaur Khalsa

COVER DESIGN & ART DIRECTOR
Ravitej Singh Khalsa

BOOK DESIGN & LAYOUT
Guru Raj Kaur Khalsa

PHOTOGRAPHY
Ravitej Singh Khalsa, Khalsa Marketing Group, Eugene, Oregon
Alan Miyataki, Toyo Miyataki Studio, Los Angeles

MODELS
Cover Model: Krishna Kaur Khalsa
Har Rai Kaur, Guru Nam Kaur, Nirinjan Kaur Khalsa, Pritham Kaur (Amelia Becker), Nicole Elliot Murray,
Amel & Elan Murray, Guru Amar Kaur Khalsa, Shanti Kaur Khalsa, Jai Kartar Kaur

PHOTO EDITORS
Nirinjan Kaur Khalsa & Ravitej Singh Khalsa

BACK COVER PHOTO OF YOGI BHAJAN
Ram Das Bir Singh Khalsa, Anaheim, California

ISBN 978-1-934532-16-4

© 2009 Kundalini Research Institute

Acknowledgements

The entire senior editorial board was instrumental in crafting this yoga manual. Their work is a tribute to the power of these teachings and the group consciousness they promote. Special thanks go to Pritpal Kaur Khalsa who researched many of the kriyas and combed through hundreds of photos to select the ones presented here. Dev Suroop Kaur and Tarn Taran Kaur dedicated a lot of time to reviewing DVDs for the sister project: *I Am a Woman: Practicing Kindness.* Hari Charn Kaur provided a steady hand and a soft touch when I needed it most. Deva Kaur's dedication to the women's teachings seems unparalleled; her encouragement and support has meant a lot throughout the course of this project. Guru Raj Kaur has been my right hand in every decision—large and small. Ravitej Singh is the man behind it all, contributing his energy and time and keen eye to making this project as beautiful as it is. Nirinjan Kaur came in at the eleventh hour to help us deliver this project on time.

Thanks to all of the models who took time out of their busy work and school schedule to help us. Two in particular put in a lot of overtime on this project, which wouldn't be as beautiful as it is without them: Guru Nam Kaur and Hari Rai Kaur. Many thanks—we couldn't have done it without you.

I Am A Woman: Creative, Sacred, & Invincible is the fruit of a beautiful tree, which has a vast network of limbs, deep roots, and a strong, sustaining trunk that is the work and dedication of the women who published the original Khalsa Women's Training Camp Notes. This book and its accompanying yoga manual, the forthcoming online lecture database of the women's teachings, and women's communities around the world are here today because of their work. We salute you and stand together to affirm: I AM A WOMAN.

SAT PURKH KAUR KHALSA, EDITOR
KUNDALINI RESEARCH INSTITUTE

About Our Cover Model

If you ever wondered whether Kundalini Yoga as taught by Yogi Bhajan® really works, we hope this picture provides a definitive answer. Krishna Kaur Khalsa is a Kundalini Yoga teacher and trainer who travels and teaches all around the world. She specializes in serving the underserved: incarcerated youth, far-reaching parts of the globe like West and Central Africa, inner city populations and rural communities here in the United States. Oh—and she celebrates her 70th birthday this year!

Donors

I Am a Woman was made possible by the generous donations of Deva Kaur Khalsa, Coral Springs, Florida.

OTHER DONORS INCLUDE:
Teresa Danton, Long Beach, California
Devi Kaur (Catherine Nedved), Webster City, Iowa
Updesh Kaur, Sunder Kaur and Inder Kaur, Yoga Village, Clearwater, Florida
Guru Atma Kaur Khalsa, Sao Paolo, Brazil
Jose Luis Dominguez Barragan, The Netherlands
Hari Datti Kaur, Cityoga, Indianapolis, Indiana
Tejtal Kaur (Marine Spring), Tuscon, Arizona
Shanti Kaur (Elizabeth Sanchez), Reseda, California
Song Gennet Lai Wan, Singapore
Nirvair Khalsa, Anchorage, Alaska
Elvira Stenson, Portland, Oregon
Mary Cline Golbitz, Bar Harbor, Maine
Barbara Marie Steinhagen, Livermore, California
Har Nal Kaur, London, United Kingdom
Maria Kalinina, Marina Del Rey, California
Marika Blossfeldt, Beacon, New York
Dawn Connelly, Seal Beach, California
Marcia Canestrano, Los Angeles, California
Ximena Hevia y Vaca, Lima, Peru
Sharlene Starr, Calgary, Canada
Calley Kuczek, Austin, Texas
Jennifer Nagel, San Antonio, Texas
Este Grobler, Woking, Surrey
Milica Apostolovic, Toronto, Canada
Noriko Snyder, Manhattan Beach, California
Eric Biese, Minneapolis, Minnesota
Linda Frank, Huntsville, Alabama
Renee Skuba, Brooklyn, New York
Siri Bani Kaur, San Rafael, California
Jay Doorek, Santa Barbara, California
Mariana Orozco, Guadalajara, Mexico
Marianne Huebner, Rochester, Minnesota
Lucille Ryan, Phoenix, Arizona
Maria Eugenia Martinez Salgado, Mexico City, Mexico
Claudia Duchene, Natlick, Massachusetts
Simeon Monov, San Jose, California
Tammy Robertson, Edmonton, Canada
Claudia Schletz, Denver, Colorado
Dharam Khalsa, Espanola, New Mexico

I Am a Woman: Creative, Sacred & Invincible

ESSENTIAL KRIYAS FOR WOMAN IN THE AQUARIAN AGE

Yogi Bhajan taught for more than 35 years here in the United States and abroad, many of those years were spent beneath the cottonwood trees of Hacienda de Guru Ram Das in Española, New Mexico, teaching specifically to women who had gathered there to study with the Master, developing their physical strength and their inner radiance, so that they could return home to serve and be a light to the world. Out of that bounty, the editors had the difficult task of selecting those kriyas, meditations and sound current practices that will serve and elevate women now and throughout the Aquarian Age. As comprehensive as this manual is, it remains just a sampling of all the technology available to women within the tradition of Kundalini Yoga as taught by Yogi Bhajan®. We hope it whets your appetite for more.

This yoga manual is the companion volume to the reader, *I Am a Woman: Creative, Sacred & Invincible* and the DVD Series *I Am a Woman: Practicing Kindness*. They work together to provide a survey of Yogi Bhajan's essential teachings for women: Part One of the reader addresses a woman's infinity, sensitivity and radiance; Part Two addresses a woman's innate power to heal herself and those around her through applied intelligence and prayer; Part Three addresses woman in polarity, those relationships and cycles that inform and transform her life; Part Four addresses a woman's physical well-being and beauty within.

The yoga manual breaks the four primary parts of the reader into 14 chapters by topic so that you can focus on a particular discipline within your own practice, generate weekend workshops for your students, or when paired in-depth with the reader, create an entire curriculum for a richer experience of the women's teachings over time. Each chapter includes a vigorous kriya or two, several meditations and a mantra or sound-current practice to connect you to the divine within you.

Our goal was to provide a primer of sorts: a way for women new to 3HO to access the core teachings of Yogi Bhajan, and a tool for teachers and trainers to present these teachings in a comprehensive and accessible way. This book will uplift you and your practice; but it is in no way meant to overwhelm you. So, if you're new to these teachings, relax. Choose one thing and excel at it. Yogi Bhajan had no patience for fanatics. He was so prolific that in fact, if you look at everything he said to do every day, it is said to take more than 48 hours to do it all. By making it impossible, he made possible the principle of self-initiation. You choose. Cultivate a practice that works with your lifestyle, be open to challenging yourself with those technologies that make you uncomfortable, come face to face with your hidden agendas, break with old patterns and habits that no longer serve you, and continually confront your weaknesses and transform them into strengths; but more than anything, be kind, to yourself and others—this is the true yoga.

Of the technologies presented, a few are specifically for women—and will have a note to that effect. The others are drawn from a wide range of lectures and classes by Yogi Bhajan, over the course of many years. Although they may not be specifically for women, they provide the tools necessary to becoming your best Self—a radiant, powerful, graceful woman.

Try everything. Think of it as a taster's menu. Even if the sound current practices seem unfamiliar and foreign, dive in. Experiment. Kundalini Yoga as taught by Yogi Bhajan® is not a path of blind faith; it is a path of experience and awareness. Awaken to your own experience, engage your sensory body, and notice the effects that a simple mantra can make in a stressful situation, or the grace that comes from listening to a *shabd* 11 times a day. These are technologies that elevate the human psyche to its excellence; they're not presented here as a form within a particular religion but rather as an expression of devotion to the Guru (wisdom) within—that same inner teacher that we tune-in to each time we open our practice with the mantra, *Ong Namo Guru Dev Namo*. Open yourself to the harmony and peace within, vibrate the cosmos, and align yourself with your Highest Self and the company of like-minded, spiritual people. In this way, you will enter the Aquarian Age with the hope of a better tomorrow and a happier today.

Combined with a close reading of the lectures and stories in the companion volume and DVD Series, we hope these teachings elevate you to your Highest Self, that you may serve the Aquarian Age with consciousness, integrity, intelligence and grace. Yogi Bhajan often said that without these teachings—the women's teachings—there would be no Aquarian Age. You, as a woman, are the key to the graceful transition from the qualities of the Piscean Age—the acquisition of power and knowledge, and the reliance on material security—to the qualities of the Aquarian Age—creativity, community, transparency, and reliance upon Infinity. This transformation calls us all to a higher level of consciousness, neutrality and shared virtues and values. Start the conversation in your own community, your own family. Begin the dialogue that will transform not only yourself and those around you, but the entire world.

Repeat the affirmation: I am a woman, I am the Grace of God and with those words bless yourself and bless the world.

SAT PURKH KAUR KHALSA
EDITOR

Table of Contents

Part One

Part Two

WOMAN IS INVINCIBLE: HEALER, LEADER, NURTURER

Part Three

SACRED FEMININE & THE DIVINE MOTHER: CREATIVE CONSCIOUSNESS & THE LONGING TO MERGE

Before You Begin

INTENTION IN PRACTICE & IN PLAY

Beginning Your Practice—Tuning-In

The practice of Kundalini Yoga as taught by Yogi Bhajan® always begins by tuning-in. This simple practice aligns your mind, your spirit and your body to become alert and assert your will so that your practice will fulfill its intention. It's a simple bowing to your Higher Self and an alignment with the teacher within. The mantra is simple but it links you to a Golden Chain of teachers, an entire body of consciousness that guides and protects your practice: *Ong Namo Guru Dev Namo. I bow to the Infinite, I bow to the Teacher within.*

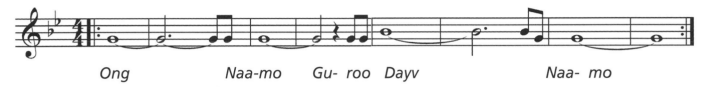

Ong   Naa-mo   Gu- roo Dayv   Naa- mo

How to End

Another tradition within Kundalini Yoga as taught by Yogi Bhajan® is a simple blessing known as *The Long Time Sun Shine song.* Sung or simply recited at the end of your practice, it allows you to dedicate your practice to all those who've preserved and delivered these teachings so that you might have the experience of your Self. It is a simple prayer to bless yourself and others. It completes the practice and allows your entire discipline to become a prayer, in service to the good of all.

May the long time sun shine upon you
All love surround you
And the pure light within you
Guide your way on.
Sat Nam.

Other Tips for a Successful Experience

Prepare for your practice by lining up all the elements that will elevate your experience: natural fiber clothing and head covering (cotton or linen), preferably white to increase your auric body; natural fiber mat, either cotton or wool; traditionally a sheep skin or other animal skin is used. If you have to use a rubber or petroleum-based mat, cover the surface with a cotton or wool blanket to protect and support your electromagnetic field. Clean air and fresh water also helps support your practice. These are ideal conditions, but in today's society, taking the time to do a simple *pranayam* at your desk or spine flex in the conference room or chanting in the kitchen while your child takes a nap can go a long way toward making your day more productive and relaxing.

Practice in Community

Kundalini Yoga cultivates group consciousness, because group consciousness is the first step toward universal consciousness, which is the goal: transcend the ego and merge with Infinity. Therefore, find a teacher in your area. Studying the science of Kundalini Yoga with a KRI certified teacher will enhance your experience and deepen your understanding of kriya, mantra, breath and posture. If there isn't a teacher in your area, consider becoming a teacher yourself. See our resources page for more information.

Find a group to practice sadhana (daily spiritual routine) with, or establish a group sadhana yourself—in your home or community center. The Aquarian Sadhana* was given by Yogi Bhajan to ground our practice now and into the Aquarian Age. Practicing with others increases the effects of sadhana exponentially. You heal others and others, in turn, heal you.

Begin Full Moon gatherings, bringing together women from all areas of life to celebrate, meditate and heal one other. Start a Peanut Hour with mothers in your neighborhood, or friends in your community, church, or workplace.

Come together as women and share your strength, ask for help when you need it, and laugh together as you participate in this game of life.

Pronunciation Guide

This simple guide to the vowel sounds in transliteration is for your convenience. More commonly used words are often spelled traditionally, for example, Sat Nam, Wahe Guru, or pranayam, even though you'll often see them written Sat Naam, Whaa-hay Guroo, and praanayaam, in order to clarify the pronunciation, especially in mantras. Gurbani is a very sophisticated sound system, and there are many other guidelines regarding consonant sounds and other rules of the language that are best conveyed through a direct student-teacher relationship. Further guidelines regarding pronunciation are available at www.kundaliniresearchinstitute.org.

a	hut
aa	mom
u	put, soot
oo	pool
i	fin
ee	feet
ai	let
ay	hay, rain
r	flick tongue on upper palate

* See *Kundalini Yoga Sadhana Guidelines*, 2nd Edition, available from the Kundalini Research Institute, for more information about creating your own sadhana and guidelines for practicing the Aquarian Sadhana.

Disclaimer

The information contained in this manual comes from ancient yogic traditions. Nothing in this manual should be construed as medical advice. Any recipes mentioned herein may contain potent herbs, botanicals and naturally occurring ingredients which have traditionally been used to support the structure and function of the human body. Always check with your personal physician or licensed health care practitioner before making any significant modification in your diet or lifestyle, to insure that the ingredients or lifestyle changes are appropriate for your personal health condition and consistent with any medication you may be taking.

Part One

WHAT IS A WOMAN?

Infinity ❀ *Divinity* ❀ *Dignity*

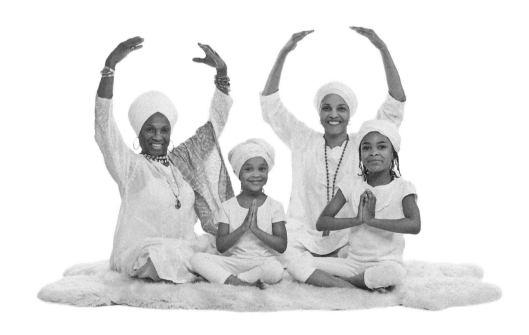

Awakening your inner vitality

ESSENTIALS FOR DAILY PRACTICE

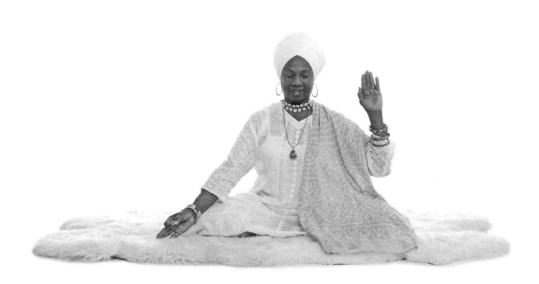

WOMAN'S INNER VITALITY is characterized by her self-esteem, her radiance, her physical glow and flow, her grace to face the challenges of life, and her practice and discipline, which brings mastery over her power as a woman. She lives in the awareness of her inherent connection with all of life—and with her own Infinity.

Living Life in Love with God

THESE DAYS WOMEN WANT INSTANT CHANGE: Help! I'm a mess! Fix me! And at every turn, woman is consistently told what is wrong with her, what needs to be "fixed," where she is not good enough. Contemporary women live in a constant state of instability and insecurity, chasing an unattainable perfection. How exhausting! Where is the happiness in that? Imagine the alternative: a woman living her life as a powerful, graceful, refined, dynamic, strong, spiritual being, constantly attuned to her inner frequency, and consistently adjusting and balancing her flow, in order to keep all systems working at their highest vibration. This most beautiful being, woman, lives her life in union with God.

A woman needs inner vitality in order to experience happiness and fulfillment. Inner vitality is characterized by her self-esteem, her radiance, her physical glow and flow, her grace to face the challenges of life, her practice and discipline, which brings mastery over her power as a woman. This woman lives in the awareness of her inherent connection with all of life—and with her own Infinity. She lives as the Spouse of God.

To live life in this way, a woman needs to make consistent, conscious choices—every day—that bring her to her own higher consciousness, and inner and outer vitality. With these consistent courageous choices, she creates a rhythm, training the mind and body to follow the soul. This is sadhana: making the choice—each and every day—to create a lifelong relationship with your soul through your daily spiritual practice.

At first sadhana can feel like you are giving something up in order to do it. It is difficult and can feel like a sacrifice. But as you progress, it becomes part of your rhythm of life; one day reaching a point where other things suddenly seem like they are getting in the way of your sadhana! When you reach this stage, you are in the state of *aradhana*.

In *aradhana*, you are declaring who the real authority is in your life. You claim your power. You work it out—and in this conquering of your own ego, your own death, you match and merge your Authentic Self with your discipline. Then you experience prabhupati and become the Spouse of God.

In *prabhupati*, and the peaceful, dynamic attunement to the flow of life, any conflict in your personality is gone. You move and your presence works; the universe co-creates with you. Then there is victory and harmony in life, even in the face of challenge or disaster.

Sadhana is a calm, serene and intelligent way of approaching our faults and defaults, our gaps and crises. Instead of the desperate action and reaction in the face of our own limitations, our own gaps—that feeling of never being enough—we face the reality: as human beings we exist in a state of "perfect imperfection." Dwell in that state; give it to God. Become the Spouse of God and rest in the embrace of your Beloved, the beauty of your own radiance, and the peace of your own soul. Every day, uplift your Self to your highest destiny, and call upon your true identity as the Grace of God. Give yourself that gift, and slowly, slowly, the steady rhythm of that identity will become the underlying core of your life, refining, balancing, steady, strong and surrendered into God's Will.

People often ask: "What is God's Will? How will I recognize it?" The answer is found in your sadhana. In sadhana, you pre-surrender to the day—and into God's Will. You align yourself, body, mind, soul, and emotion, all moving in the same direction. Sadhana is a discipline of the mind and body to serve the soul. It's as if your consciousness were asking, "Let's get this human incarnation straight, shall we?" If a woman sets her intention each day to be the Spouse of God, to live as *prabhupati*, life flows—challenges and all.

Sadhana is a victory, a way of living which conquers your low self-esteem, your self-sabotage. It is a victory of your commitment to your higher Self over your insecurity and fear, that part of you that still believes you're small. To live as a graceful, powerful woman—this commitment to consciousness is the key to your inner vitality.

Treasure of Technology

In the pages of this manual you will find a treasure of technologies for cultivating inner vitality and grace. They are yours to incorporate into your daily practice. In this first section we offer some of the principle technologies that many women have brought into their daily lives, to develop a core experience of strength and intuition.

SADHANA
Daily spiritual practice training body and mind to serve the soul

ARADANA
Your individual self becomes one with the Universal Self

PRABHUPATI
Living as the Spouse of God

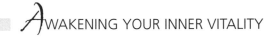

40-Day Sadhana

"There are two guiding instincts in a human. He is either improving his future or blocking his future improvement. If you are conscious of this, and have an honest and sincere urge to improve the future, you will always have promoting habits. If you cannot care for God, at least care for the future."

—Yogi Bhajan

To master the effects of a meditation, practice it as a sadhana, a daily discipline. This will develop life-promoting habits, or patterns. Habits control us to such an extent that it is said that we can actually change our destiny by changing our habits. According to the science of yoga, the human mind works in cycles. We can use those cycles to help replace unwanted patterns of behavior (mental or emotional habits), with new, more positive ones. For example, committing to a particular meditation or kriya for a specific period of time:

> 40 days to change a pattern;
> 90 days to confirm the pattern;
> 120 days, the new patterns is who you are;
> 1,000 days, you have mastered the new pattern.

A 40-day practice allows the meditation to provoke your subconscious to release any thoughts and emotional patterns that hinder you. A good meditation will break your old patterns, clear the subconscious and plant the seed for a new pattern. Try to meditate at the same time each day. It is also helpful to keep a journal of your daily practice, to witness your own process.

The Aquarian Sadhana

Part of the 3HO lifestyle, and side-by-side with any personal practice, is the core, morning sadhana that was given by Yogi Bhajan, known as the Aquarian Sadhana, practiced every morning during the *amrit vela* or Nectar Time. You can find out about this practice, and how to join in, from any Kundalini Yoga Teacher.

Yogic scriptures call for at least two-and-a-half hours of sadhana before the rising of the sun. This is determined by the law of karma: everything you give, you receive back tenfold. So if you dedicate one-tenth of each day to your higher consciousness, your whole day is covered by the returning energy.

Sadhana before sunrise is recommended because the angle of the Sun to the Earth at that time is very effective for meditation. Also there is so much *prana* during these early hours, and the body's rhythms support physical cleansing more than any other time of the day. Few people are awake and busy, so the clutter and bustle of daily activities does not interfere with your practice. Those of us who have risen during the *amrit vela* for years often joke that "God can hear you better because no one else is awake."

Group Sadhana

There is a special power to doing the Aquarian Sadhana in a group. Yogi Bhajan taught that the progression for developing one's spiritual consciousness is threefold: individual consciousness, through group consciousness, will bring you to Infinite consciousness. With group sadhana, we support our individual commitment while dwelling in a sacred space that supports one another in the consistent, conscious choice for higher consciousness.

A person once asked Yogi Bhajan about sadhana.

They said, "I thought that once sadhana is done, nothing should happen to you."

Yogi Bhajan replied: "No, when sadhana happens, everything should happen to you, and you should come out as a winner, you should come out victorious! That is what sadhana gives you. It doesn't give you a written guarantee from God. The one who does sadhana builds in himself such a powerful personality, he can conquer anything! That is why I do my own sadhana. I have been doing it for years—I do it even now. Some people ask me, 'You are a Master, why do you do sadhana?' I say, 'To remain a Master!'"

GURU RAJ KAUR KHALSA
VANCOUVER, B.C. CANADA

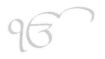

JAPJI SAHIB AND THE SHABD GURU
Song of the Soul

"Give because God gives to you. Love because that is your purpose in life. Shine because it is important. Share because it is demanded of you. How can you do it? In Japji, Guru Nanak gave you guidance, telling you the way he found liberation, 'In the ambrosial hour, meditate on the True Identity. Your karma will be covered, and you will see the door of liberation.'"

– Yogi Bhajan, May 2, 2000

These days, many people are having spontaneous spiritual experiences. The souls of so many are opening up, ready to understand and embrace life in more subtle and profound ways. But in the middle of our still imbalanced world, what do we do with these experiences? Ancient spiritual traditions teach us that we need a guide of some kind, a Guru. A Guru is a conscious being who has already walked the path of spiritual awakening and can take us, step by step, along the way, protecting us from the pitfalls of illusion and ego. Yet, with so many spiritual teachers today, it is difficult to know who to follow.

Many years ago, I moved to Española, New Mexico, to study with the Kundalini Yoga Master, Yogi Bhajan. Yogi Bhajan did not allow me to relate to him as a Guru. Rather, he took our relationship of Teacher and student and used it as a way to teach me about the Shabd Guru. But how to explain the Shabd Guru? It requires taking a step back to see the big picture of life, death and rebirth.

We are not who we think we are, and we are not here for the reasons our minds tell us. We are the Spirit of the Divine and we have come into form to enjoy the experience of creation, of being alive. We have come in many different forms, over thousands of different lifetimes, to enjoy creation from a myriad of perspectives. Every time we are born in one form or another, we forget where we came from and become absorbed in the play of creation. But this forgetfulness, when it comes to being human, can create difficulties. The human consciousness is so subtle, so sophisticated, it was made to understand itself as a manifestation of Divine Light. But there is so much to learn and experience in the human form, sometimes we can get lost. Between the process of forgetting where we came from and the process of feeling all these human sensations, we get trapped into forgetting what our True Identity really is.

Realizing this problem, the Creator developed different spiritual paths, disciplines and practices—dharmas—as short cuts to mastering the human experience. Through dharma, spiritual practice, we learn the essential lessons much more quickly so that we can begin living the reality of our own Divinity. Dharma is born of the compassion of the Creator, and like all natural organic systems on Earth, dharma expresses itself in more than one form, in more than one culture, in more than one way. There are many different kinds of tomatoes. But they are all good to eat. There are many different paths of awakening. But they are all going to take you there. It is a question of what your soul needs.

MORE THAN 500 YEARS AGO, a beautiful man was born, in what is now India, who understood this truth. His name was Guru Nanak. He spent most of his youth studying with spiritual teachers and practitioners of every tradition known in his day. He saw the Divine Light in everyone and believed that our common brotherhood and sisterhood was the highest spiritual reality. In his early 30s, Guru Nanak had his own enlightenment experience. In that state of ecstasy, Guru Nanak sang a song—that song is known as *Japji Sahib*, the Song of the Soul—and *Japji Sahib* is a manifestation of the Shabd Guru.

The Power to Heal and Transform

Japji Sahib works on two levels. First, it offers beautiful instructions about how to understand life, the universe and your own place in this vast cosmic play. In this way, it operates on the level of language and meaning. But as a manifestation of the Shabd Guru, it also has a powerful effect on another level entirely. The sounds of the words, themselves, have the capacity to heal and transform your physical, mental, emotional and spiritual reality. As you chant the words, a powerful alchemy takes place. Your body, like an instrument, begins to vibrate at the same level of consciousness that Guru Nanak was in when he had his enlightenment experience. As that vibration continues, anything within you—your karmas, your subconscious, your habits—which does not match that high frequency starts to "shake loose." As you keep chanting in the frequency of Universal Consciousness, you begin to clear and remove your own blocks to experiencing Universal Consciousness. This is a process between you, your breath, and the sound current of the Shabd Guru. No other person has the power to intercede. As you chant, you purify yourself; and in this way, the Shabd Guru guides you, in time and through grace, to merge into your Infinite Identity.

We are moving into an Age in which humanity will perceive reality as a flow of information. Our survival will depend on how we flow with that information. The Shabd Guru is a Guru that teaches, through the Sound Current, how to flow with the most subtle information of all: the creative command of the Divine, which is continually creating the creation and bringing us to ever deeper and vaster realms of awareness.

Guru Nanak founded Sikh Dharma in two ways: he offered a truly universal and inclusive vision of the human race; and he laid down a specific path through the technology of the Shabd Guru. Within the teachings of *Japji Sahib* is not only a description of how to see the Divine, but also the path of how to be Divine, through vibrating the Sound Current—and this is its great power and sublime secret.

May you be blessed unto Infinity and may the journey of your own soul take to you your highest truth. May the remembrance that the Creator set you here for a purpose awaken you to live in the purity of your own genuineness of spirit. May you ever be blessed to live healthy, happy and holy.

EK ONG KAAR KAUR KHALSA
ESPAÑOLA, NEW MEXICO

EK ONG KAR SAT NAM KARTA PURKH NIRBHO NIRVAIR AKAL MOORAT AJUNI
SAIBHANG GUR PRASAD JAP! AD SACH JUGAD SACH HAIBI SACH NANAK HOSI BHI SACH

THE **MAGNIFICENT NINE**

1. **Cat Stretch**. Lying on the back, stretch the arms above the head on the ground. Keeping the shoulders on the ground, bend one knee over onto the ground of the opposite side of the body. Do the same with the other leg.

2. **Eye Opener**. Lying flat, place the palms tightly over closed eyes. Open the eyes, and look directly into the palms. Holding the gaze, slowly lift the hands to 18 inches above the face. Bring the fingertips down to the center of the forehead, and massage with a circular motion, out to the temples and down both sides of the face to the tip of the chin. Massage your nose and ears, squeeze the nostrils and ear lobes.

3. **Stretch Pose**. Lie on the back with the feet together, toes pointed. Flatten the lower back. Place hands palms down over the thighs, pointing towards the toes. Lift the head up, apply Neck Lock and look at the toes. Lift the feet up 6 inches and begin Breath of Fire for **10 to 15 seconds**.

4. **Cobra Pose**. Lying on the stomach, place hands under the shoulders with palms flat. Elongate the spine, lift the chest and heart up, drop the shoulders, and stretch the head back. Straighten the arms. Long Deep Breathing or Breath of Fire for **1 minute**.

5. **Cat-Cow**. On the hands and knees, hands are shoulder-width apart, fingers facing forward, knees directly under the hips. Inhale and tilt the pelvis forward, arching the spine down, head and neck stretched up. Exhale and tilt the pelvis the opposite way, arching the spine up, pressing chin to chest. Breathe powerfully. Speed can be increased as flexibility is gained. **3 minutes**.

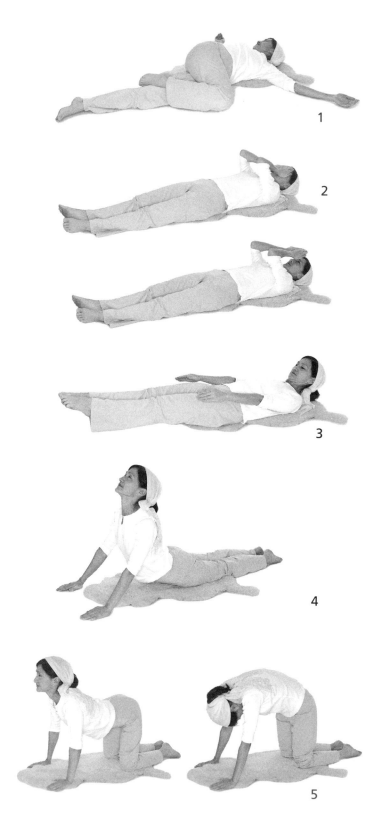

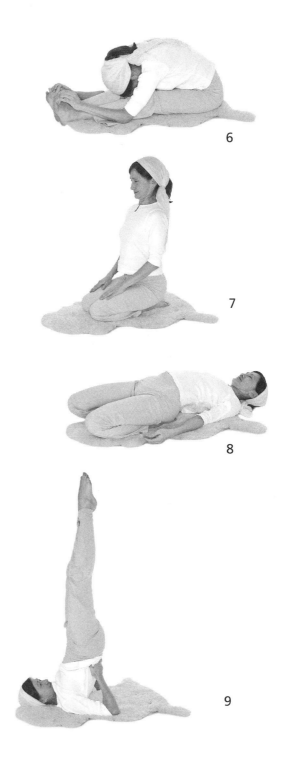

6. **Front Stretch**. Sitting down, stretch the legs out in front. Grab the big toes in finger-lock. Inhale, lengthen the spine. Exhale, bend forward bringing chest to thighs, and nose to knees. Avoid leading with the head. Do this three times a day, to check your mental strength.

"Anytime you feel tense, your energy is off, you need to balance it, and you want to face the world for hours, do this exercise. Do it every four hours. For a female, this is a must! Make it your 'Mental Standard.'"

7. **Rock Pose**. Sit on the heels with palms flat on the thighs. Do Breath of Fire or Long Deep Breathing for **5 minutes**.

8. **Fish Pose**. From Rock Pose, keeping knees bent, and the feet outside the hips, extend the torso back until the head and shoulders rest on the ground. Hold for **5 to 7 minutes**.

"Whenever you eat, you must sit on your heels for 5 to 7 minutes. If it is possible for you in the evening, in the twilight zone, when the sun is setting, lie down like this flat on your back. If a woman can do this, she will seldom get sick. Do this for 5 to 7 minutes."

9. **Shoulder Stand**. From lying on the back, place the hands on the hips, just below the waist, and bring the hips and legs up to a vertical position, spine and legs perpendicular to the ground. Support the weight of the body on the elbows and shoulders using the hands to support the lower spine. The chin is pressed into the chest. Hold for **5 minutes** in the morning.

Shoulder Stand is especially good for the female. It releases pressure on all the organs and stimulates the thyroid gland.

About This Kriya

These nine exercises were recommended by Yogi Bhajan in 1988 as a daily practice for every woman to maintain her youth and beauty. *Note: Some may remember this as originally called "The Magnificent Seven." In those days, that was the name of a popular movie. Some of the postures had been coupled together to appear as 7 instead of 9.*

SAT KRIYA
AN ESSENTIAL KRIYA OF KUNDALINI YOGA

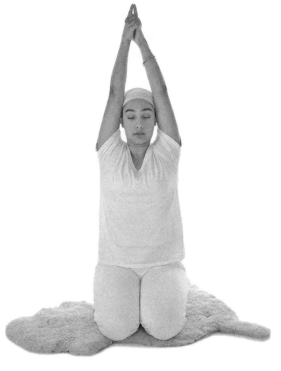

POSTURE: Sit on the heels in Rock Pose, knees together. Stretch the arms over the head with elbows straight, until the arms hug the sides of the head. Interlace all the fingers except the index fingers. Men cross the right thumb over the left. Women cross the left thumb over the right. The spine stays still and straight. This is neither a spinal flex nor a pelvic thrust. Remain firmly seated on the heels throughout the motions of the kriya.

MANTRA & RHYTHM: Begin to chant *Sat Nam* with a constant rhythm of about 8 times per 10 seconds. As you pull the navel in and up toward the spine, chant *Sat* from the Navel Point. Feel it as a pressure from the Third Chakra. With the sound *Naam*, relax the belly.

As you continue in a steady rhythm, the root and diaphragm locks are automatically pulled. The steady waves of effort from the navel gradually enlist the movement of the greater abdomen. The force is through the navel but the two locks come along sympathetically. This natural pull of the two locks creates a physiological balance. Blood pressure is maintained evenly. The rhythmic contraction and relaxation produces waves of energy that circulate, energize, and heal the body.

The focus of the sound *Naam* can be either at the Navel Point or at the Brow Point (the point where the eyebrows meet at the root of the nose; the area that corresponds to the Sixth Chakra).

BREATH: The breath regulates itself—no breath focus is necessary.

TIME: Continue for **3 to 31 minutes.**

TO END: Inhale and gently squeeze the muscles from the buttocks all the way up along the spine. Hold it briefly as you concentrate on the area just above the top of the head. Then exhale completely. Inhale, exhale totally and hold the breath out as you apply a firm *mahabandh*—contract the lower pelvis, lift the diaphragm, lock in the chin, and squeeze all the muscles from the buttocks up to the neck. Hold the breath out for 5 to 20 seconds according to your comfort and capacity. Inhale. Relax. If you practice this as a complete kriya in itself, the relaxation is ideally twice the length of time as you practiced the Sat Kriya. (If practiced as part of a *kriya*, follow the relaxation times specified.)

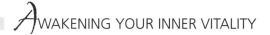

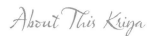
About This Kriya

Sat Kriya is essential to the practice of Kundalini Yoga. It is one of the few exercises that is a complete kriya in itself—an action or series of actions that completes a process and has a predictable outcome.

As a kriya, it is a process that works on all levels of your being—known and unknown—making you more capable of responding to your own subtlety and totality. Approached with patience, steadiness, and moderation, the end result is assured. If you have very little time and you wish to do a beautiful practice, make this kriya part of your daily routine.

One of the primary actions is to balance the energies of the lower triangle of chakras, the energy distribution centers, by mixing the *prana* and *apana* at the navel center. This generates a heat in the system and opens the inner channels to the upward flow and rotation of energy. The contraction of the navel and the gentle, automatic pull of the *mulbandh* guide the forward projection and mixing of the chakra energies. It is excellent for digestive troubles and for transcending fears. The excellence of Sat Kriya is that all three lower chakras are pulled together and act in unison. The correlated action of all three centers multiplies the effect and stabilizes the changes.

Sat Kriya tones the nervous system, calms emotional disarray, and channels creative and sexual energies of the body. The entire sexual system is stimulated and strengthened. It relaxes and releases many phobias about sexual behavior, potency, and capacity.

The most common errors when doing Sat Kriya are to pull too strongly from the base, with a heavily squeezed *mulbandh*, or to lift the arms too strongly, which squeezes the Diaphragm Lock (*udiyana bandh*) while ignoring the lower body. The goal is a balance: pull from the Navel Point, and as the Navel Point is pulled the *mulbandh* tightens, followed closely and seamlessly by the Diaphragm Lock. As those locks are applied, the chest lifts and a natural Neck Lock results. The arms stay fully extended, the main movement is in the torso, the spine and abdomen. The spine stays straight and does not flex, as one would do in the Kundalini Yoga posture, Spine Flex. The power comes from the natural rhythm and wave of energy initiated with *Sat* at the navel and released with *Naam*.

The subtle blending of the *prana* and *apana* is accomplished with each repetition of the mantra. The *bij* mantra itself establishes a *sattvic* quality of neutrality and stillness at the navel, which allows the kundalini to flow naturally, in proportion to the individual need, for physical, mental and spiritual clarity and healing.

BUILDING THE PRACTICE GRADUALLY:
In the beginning practice Sat Kriya for just 3 minutes. Give your attention to perfecting the form, rhythm, and concentration. To build it up in time and effect, start with rotation cycles: 3 minutes of Sat Kriya with 2 minutes of relaxation. Repeat this cycle 3 to 5 times. Build gradually. Then switch the cycles to 5 minutes Sat Kriya and 5 minutes rest. Then add 3 to 5 minutes as you are comfortable and accomplished. Soon you will be able to do the entire 31 minutes.

COMMON MISTAKES
Lifting the shoulders as if doing a shoulder shrug.
Moving the torso as in spinal flex rather than fixing the spine straight and letting the motion come from the navel area.
Accelerating or varying the speed of the rhythm.
Lowering the pitch rather than keeping it steady.

ALTERNATE SEATED POSTURE
Though the effects will not be as strong or precise, if physically unable to sit on the heels, Sat Kriya can be done in Easy Pose.

ALTERNATE MUDRA
One may have the palms flat, rather than interlaced fingers. This is a more advanced version of the posture.

SODARSHAN CHAKRA KRIYA

DECEMBER 1990

POSTURE: Sit in Easy Pose with a straight spine, and a light Neck Lock.

EYE FOCUS: Eyes are fixed at the tip of the nose.

MUDRA, MANTRA & BREATH PATTERN:
a) Block the right nostril with the right thumb. Inhale slowly and deeply through the left nostril. Suspend the breath. Mentally chant the mantra *Wahe Guru* 16 times:

WHAA-HAY GUROO

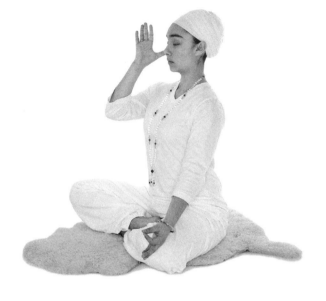

Pump the Navel Point 3 times with each repetition, once on **WHAA**; once on **HAY**; and once on **GUROO**, for a total of 48 unbroken pumps.

b) After the 16 repetitions, unblock the right nostril. Place the right index finger (pinkie finger can also be used) to block off the left nostril, and exhale slowly and deeply through the right nostril.

Continue in this pattern.

TIME: 3-31 minutes. Master practitioners may steadily develop this practice to **62 minutes**, to a maximum of **2 1/2 hours** a day.

TO END: Inhale, hold the breath 5-10 seconds, then exhale. Stretch the arms up and shake every part of your body for *1 minute*, so the energy can spread.

About This Meditation

This is one of the greatest meditations you can practice. It has considerable transformational powers. The personal identity is rebuilt, giving the individual a new perspective on the Self. It retrains the mind. According to the *Tantra Shastras*, it is said it can purify your past karma and the subconscious impulses that may block you from fulfilling you. It balances all the 27 facets of life and mental projections, and gives you the pranic power of health and healing. It establishes inner happiness and a state of flow and ecstasy in life. It opens your inner universe to relate, co-create, and complete the external universe.

Treat the practice with reverence and increase your depth, dimension, caliber, and happiness. It gives you a new start against all odds.

"Of all the 20 types of yoga, including Kundalini Yoga, this is the highest kriya. This meditation cuts through all darkness. It will give you a new start. It is the simplest kriya, but at the same time the hardest. It cuts through all barriers of the neurotic or psychotic inside-nature. When one is in a very bad state, techniques imposed from the outside will not work. The pressure has to be stimulated from within. The tragedy of life is when the subconscious releases garbage into the conscious mind. This kriya invokes the Kundalini to give you the necessary vitality and intuition to combat the negative effects of the subconscious mind.

There is no time, no place, no space, and no condition attached to this mantra. Each garbage point has its own time to clear. If you are going to clean your own garbage, you must estimate and clean it as fast or as slow as you want. Start practicing slowly— the slower the better. "

— Yogi Bhajan

KIRTAN KRIYA
CARRYING US THROUGH THE AQUARIAN AGE

This kriya is one of three that Yogi Bhajan mentioned would carry us through the Aquarian Age, even if all other teachings were lost. There are four principle components to practicing Kirtan Kriya correctly: Mantra, Mudra, Voice, and Visualization.

POSTURE: Sit in Easy Pose with a straight spine, and a light Neck Lock.

EYE FOCUS: Focus at the Brow Point.

MANTRA: This *kriya* uses the five primal sounds, or the *Panj Shabd*— *S, T, N, M, A*—in the original *bij* (seed) form of the mantra *Sat Nam*:

SAA — *Infinity, cosmos, beginning*
TAA — *Life, existence*
NAA — *Death, change, transformation*
MAA — *Rebirth*

This is the cycle of creation. From the Infinite comes life and individual existence. From life comes death or change. From death comes the rebirth of consciousness. From rebirth comes the joy of the Infinite through which compassion leads back to life. Chant the '*A*' like 'mom,' in the following manner:

SAA TAA NAA MAA

Each repetition of the entire mantra takes 3 to 4 seconds.

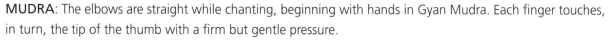

SAA   TAA   NAA   MAA

MUDRA: The elbows are straight while chanting, beginning with hands in Gyan Mudra. Each finger touches, in turn, the tip of the thumb with a firm but gentle pressure.

SAA — *Press the Jupiter (index) finger and thumb.*
TAA — *Press the Saturn (middle) finger and thumb.*
NAA — *Press the Sun (ring) finger and thumb.*
MAA — *Press the Mercury (pinkie) finger and thumb.*

Begin again with the index finger.

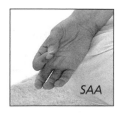
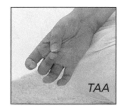
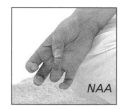
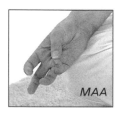

VOICE

The mantra is chanted in the three languages of consciousness:

Aloud (the voice of the human)	—	awareness of the things of the world
Whisper (the voice of the lover)	—	experiencing the longing to belong
Silent (the voice of the divine)	—	meditate on Infinity or mentally vibrate

VISUALIZATION

Visualize the flow of the sounds in an "L" form. As you meditate feel there is a constant inflow of cosmic energy into your solar center (Tenth Gate, the Crown Chakra). As the energy enters the top of the head, you flow the sounds *Sa, Ta, Na, Ma* through. As you chant *SAA* for example, the "*S*" starts at the top of the head and the "*A*" moves down and out through the Brow Point, projected to Infinity. This energy flow follows the energy pathway called the Golden Cord—the connection between the pineal and pituitary gland. Some people may occasionally experience headaches from practicing Kirtan Kriya if they do not use this "L" form. The most common reason for this is improper circulation of *prana* in the solar centers.

TO BEGIN THE PRACTICE

Sit straight in Easy Pose and meditate at the Brow Point.

Chant aloud for 5 minutes.

Then whisper for 5 minutes.

Then go deeply into silence, mentally vibrating the sound for 10 minutes.

Then whisper for 5 minutes.

Then chant aloud for 5 minutes.

TO END: Close the meditation with a deep inhale and suspend the breath as long as comfortable—up to a minute—relaxing it smoothly to complete **1 minute of absolute stillness and silence**. Then, stretch the hands up as far as possible and spread the fingers wide. Stretch the spine and take several deep breaths. Relax.

About This Meditation

Practicing this meditation brings a total mental balance to the individual psyche. As you vibrate on each fingertip, you alternate your electrical polarities. The index and ring fingers are electrically negative, relative to the other fingers. This causes a balance in the electro-magnetic projection of the aura. If during the silent part of the meditation your mind wanders uncontrollably, go back to a whisper, to a loud voice, to a whisper and back into silence. Do this as often as necessary to stay alert.

Each time the mudra is closed by joining the thumb with a finger, the ego "seals" the effect of that mudra in the consciousness. The effects are as follows:

SIGN	FINGER	NAME	EFFECT
Jupiter	Index	Gyan Mudra	Knowledge
Saturn	Middle	Shuni Mudra	Wisdom, intelligence, patience
Sun	Ring	Surya Mudra	Vitality, energy of life
Mercury	Pinkie	Buddhi Mudra	Ability to communicate

Practicing this meditation is both a science and an art. It is an art in the way it molds consciousness and the refinement of sensation and insight it produces. It is a science in the tested certainty of the results it produces. This meditation is based on the tested experience of many people, in many conditions, over many years. It is based on the structure of the psyche and the laws of action and reaction that accompany each sound, movement and posture. Chanting the *Panj Shabd*—the primal or nuclear form of *Sat Nam*—has profound energy within it because we are breaking the *bij* (seed or atom) of the sound into its primary elements.

The timing can be decreased or increased as long as you maintain the ratio of spoken, whispered, and silent chanting—always end with **1 minute of complete stillness and silence**. Yogi Bhajan has said that a person who wears pure white and meditates on this sound current for 2-1/2 hours a day for one year, will know the Unknown and see the Unseen. Through this constant practice, the mind awakens to the infinite capacity of the soul for sacrifice, service, and creation.

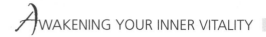

GRACE OF GOD MEDITATION

PART ONE

POSTURE: Lie on the back, fully relaxing the face and body.

EYE FOCUS: The eyes are closed.

MANTRA: *I AM GRACE OF GOD*

Inhale deeply, hold the breath in while silently repeating the mantra **10 times**. Tense the fingers one at a time to keep count.

Exhale all the air out, hold it out and repeat the mantra **10 times**.

Continue this process of repeating the mantra **10 times on each inhale** and **10 times on each exhale**, for a total of **5 inhalations** and **5 exhalations**. This totals **100 silent repetitions**.

PART TWO

POSTURE: Relax your breath, and with eyes still closed, slowly come sitting up into Easy Pose.

MUDRA: Bring the right hand into Gyan Mudra, resting on the knee. The left hand is held up at the level of the left shoulder, palm flat and facing forward, as if you are taking an oath.

BREATH & MOVEMENT: Keep the breath relaxed and normal. Tense only one finger of the left hand at a time, keeping the other fingers straight but relaxed. Meditate on the governing energy of each finger *(see table)*, then repeat the mantra aloud **5 times**.

   Beginning with the Mercury Finger, continue this sequence for each of the remaining fingers, finishing with the thumb.

TO END: Relax and meditate silently for a few minutes.

GOVERNING ENERGY OF EACH FINGER			
Little Finger	MERCURY	Power to relate & communicate, subconscious communication with self	WATER
Ring Finger	SUN & VENUS	Physical health, vitality, grace, and beauty	FIRE
Middle Finger	SATURN	Channel emotion to devotion & patience	AIR
Index Finger	JUPITER	Wisdom and expansion, open space for change	ETHER
Thumb		Positive ego	EARTH

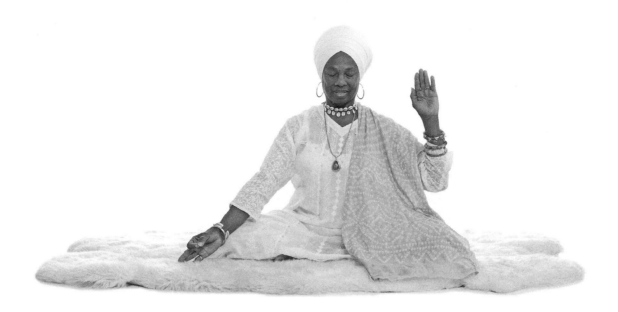

About This Meditation

It is said that when a woman practices this meditation for one year, her aura will become tipped with gold or silver, and great strength and God's healing powers will flow through her. Positive affirmation is an age-old technology. Words increase in power through repetition, and when you are repeating truth, the impact is enormous. Yogi Bhajan gave us this meditation, which is one of the most powerful affirmations a woman can do. The fact is, woman *is* the Grace of God. Woman is Shakti. The problem is, she doesn't know it.

This meditation is designed to evoke and manifest the inner grace, strength, and radiance of each woman. It helps her to tune in directly with the Adi Shakti, the Primal Power within her own being. It empowers a woman to channel her emotions in a positive direction, strengthen her weaknesses, develop mental clarity and effective communication, and give her the patience to go through the tests of her own karma. It enables her to merge the limited ego into Divine Will, as well as to improve her physical health.

By practicing this meditation, a woman's thoughts, behavior, personality, and projection become aligned with the Infinite beauty and nobility unveiled by the mantra. It balances the five elements. The amazing thing is, this is such an easy meditation to do! You might pass it over because it is so simple and not realize what a profound effect it can have on your life.

Practice it faithfully, twice a day for 40 days. It is recommended for women going through menopause to practice it 5 times a day.

Best to practice on an empty stomach.

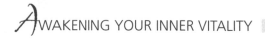

KUNDALINI BHAKTI MEDITATION
Adi Shakti Namo Namo

This devotional mantra (a Bhakti mantra), invokes the primary Creative Power which is manifest as the feminine. It calls upon the Mother Power. It will help you to be free of the insecurities which block freedom of action. By meditating on it one can obtain a deeper understanding of the constant interplay between the manifest and the unmanifest qualities of the cosmos and consciousness.

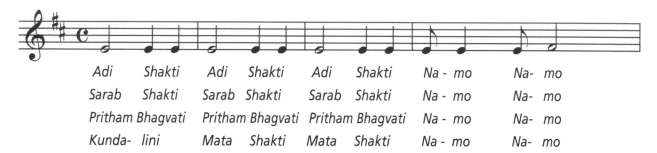

Adi	Shakti	Adi	Shakti	Adi	Shakti	Na-mo	Na-mo
Sarab	Shakti	Sarab	Shakti	Sarab	Shakti	Na-mo	Na-mo
Pritham Bhagvati		Pritham Bhagvati		Pritham Bhagvati		Na-mo	Na-mo
Kunda-lini		Mata	Shakti	Mata	Shakti	Na-mo	Na-mo

I bow to the Primal Power.
I bow to the all Encompassing Power and Energy.
I bow to that through which God creates.
I bow to the creative power of the kundalini, the Divine Mother Power.

A WOMAN'S PERSONAL MANTRA AS AN ESSENTIAL DAILY PRACTICE
This powerful mantra belongs to all women to call upon any time. She can chant it freely and powerfully at will, any time.

WITH CELESTIAL COMMUNICATION
This mantra can be experiencing powerfully by adding Celestial Communication. Celestial Communication is mudra in motion. A tool for mental relaxation, it is meditation with mantra and movement of the arms and upper body. The meaning of the mantra is expressed through movement. The mantra will move the spirit, and at the same time, the head and feelings will be heard. Yogi Bhajan describes its impact:

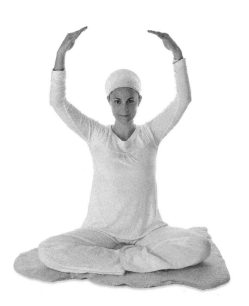

"Everything comes from stress. If you want to get rid of this inner-grown stress, here is one solution. There's no power more than the power of the word, and when the word is formed through the body, the entire being is purified, relaxed..."

You can create your own Celestial Communiction movements, or learn already developed sequences.

WITH SPECIFIC MEDITATIONS
Yogi Bhajan taught this mantra with several meditations, such as in Adi Shakti Meditation for Vitality on page 126, and Meditation to Call on the Divine Mother on page 143.

SENSITIVITY

CONNECT TO YOUR ETERNAL POWER

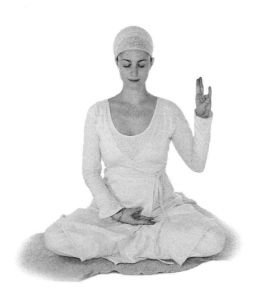

A WOMAN uses her sensitivity not to confront or compete but to bring to zero—*shuniya*—and from that emptiness, through her compassion, her kindness, and her intelligence, she creates the things she wants.

I am a Woman, I am the Grace of God

As a woman I rely on my intuition and my sensitivity to command the Earth. It is through a calm and open heart, a clear meditative and projective mind, that we can connect the Heavens to the Earth and live in grace and nobility. A woman loses when she competes on the Earth; she wins when she brings the Heavens down to the Earth, this is her eternal power.

A woman has two Arclines: ear-to-ear across the Third Eye and nipple-to-nipple across the Heart Center. The Arcline at the brow represents the destiny—and the actions that fulfill that destiny. The Arcline at the Heart Center represents relationships and a woman's ability to empathize and project compassion. Because she has this second Arcline, she has a tremendous capacity to create the other. She has access to a process in relationships that sees beyond the surface; she intuits and understands not only the conscious but also the subconscious and unconscious relays. When a woman merges these two capacities—these two Arclines—she has tremendous creativity to plant a seed, nourish it, and create reality, her projected reality. A woman uses her sensitivity to nurture, protect, surround, beam, and create the future through her projection.

A woman is always both a woman and a mother. Each role has its own capacities and duties. A woman uses her sensitivity not to confront or compete but to bring to zero—*shuniya*—and from that emptiness, through her compassion, her kindness, and her intelligence, she creates the things she wants. Create prosperity. A mother uses her sensitivity to protect, nurture, and support her environments so that anything she applies her creativity to, succeeds.

THE KRIYAS AND MEDITATIONS IN THIS SECTION were selected to support you in being centered on the Earth and accessing the Heavens. The **Kriya for the Instinctual Self** creates balance in the pelvic area and the lower chakras to allow us to walk in balance on the Earth and be constant and consistent. The **Meditation to Remember the Heavens** makes your mind clear so that as a woman you can connect to the heavens, using the body and the breath to deliver the experience of reverence and respect of the Earth and the Heavens. **The Calm and Open Heart Kriya** clears your mind to allow you to live in your heart. **Beaming and Creating the Future** gives you the opportunity to practice the art of connecting these two Arclines and projecting the reality you want. **The Mercury Projection Meditation** incorporates the power of your communication to refine and clarify your projection.

Finally, **The Song of Victory:** *I-aanree-ay*, a *shabd* practice, gives you an opportunity to meditate on your virtues, to acknowledge your place in the world, and to realize your destiny as the soul bride. Sensitivity, like everything, has a polarity—strength and weakness. Using the sound current of the Shabd Guru allows you to plug into the highest consciousness and highest destiny of yourself as a woman; and delivers you from the subconscious fears and insecurities, the emotions and commotions that limit your capacity to create from a neutral, elevated space.

Use your sensitivity wisely and you will never fail as a woman.

I am a Woman, I am the Grace of God.

HARI CHARN KAUR KHALSA
ESPAÑOLA, NEW MEXICO

KRIYA FOR THE INSTINCTUAL SELF

1. **Butterfly Pose**. Sit with the soles of the feet pressed together. Grab the feet with both hands and draw them into the groin, keeping the knees as close to the floor as possible. Inhale and flex the spine forward. Exhale and flex the spine back. Head stays straight. Continue with a steady rhythm, coordinating the movement with the breath for **I to 3 minutes**. Inhale and hold the breath briefly. Exhale and relax. *This exercise loosens the lower spine and stimulates the flow of sexual energy.*

2. **Cobra Pose**. Lying on the stomach, place hands under the shoulders with palms flat. Elongate the spine, lift the chest and heart up, drop the shoulders, and stretch the head back. Straighten the arms gradually, without straining.

   (a) Inhale and raise the buttocks so that the body forms a straight line from the head to the heels.

   (b) Exhale and lower the body back into Cobra Pose. Continue rhythmically with powerful breathing for **1 to 3 minutes**. Then inhale in Cobra Pose, suspend the breath briefly, apply *mulbandh*. Exhale and relax. *This exercise works to strengthen the lower back and to balance the flow of sexual energy with the region of the Third Chakra.*

3. **Crow Pose**. Crouch down into Crow Pose, with the soles of the feet flat on the floor, and the knees wide, drawn into the chest. Keep the spine as straight as possible. Wrap the arms around the knees with the fingers interlocked in Venus Lock. Begin Breath of Fire. Continue for **1 to 3 minutes**. Inhale. Exhale and relax. *This exercise circulates the energy of the lower three chakras and opens up the circulation to the hips and lower intestines.*

4. **Leg Lifts**. Lie on the back. Inhale and raise both legs up to 90 degrees. Exhale and lower the legs. Continue with powerful breathing and a steady rhythm for **1 to 3 minutes**. *This exercise strengthens the abdomen, setting the Navel Point and balancing prana and apana.*

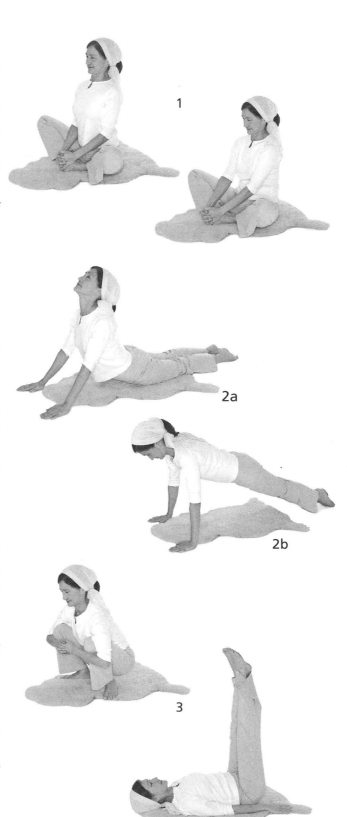

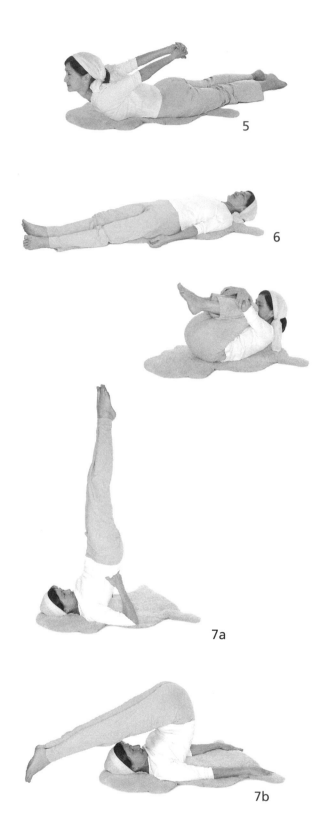

5

6

7a

7b

5. **Modified Boat Pose**. Lie on the stomach. Interlock the fingers in Venus Lock at the small of the back. Inhale, raising the head and stretching the arms as far up as possible. Begin Breath of Fire. Continue for **1 to 3 minutes**. Inhale. Exhale and relax.

This exercise strengthens the lower back. allows the energy to flow to the mid-spine and opens the nerve channels in the area of the solar plexus.

6. Relax on the back for **1 to 3 minutes** with the arms at the sides and the palms facing up. Then, pull the knees to the chest, wrap the arms around the knees, press the the head forward, nose towards the knees. Rock back and forth on the spine from the base to the top and back for **1 minute**.

This period of relaxation and the exercise following it, relax the spine and distribute the energy from the previous exercises.

7. **Shoulder Stand**. Lying on the back, place the hands on the hips, just below the waist. Bring the hips and legs up to a vertical position, making the spine and legs perpendicular to the ground. Support the weight of the body on the elbows and shoulders using the hands to support the lower spine. The chin is pressed into the chest.

(a) Begin Breath of Fire in this position. Continue for **1 to 3 minutes**.

(b) **Plow Pose**. Continuing Breath of Fire, come into Plow Pose, by carefully bending at the waist, dropping the legs down and touching the pointed toes on the ground behind the head. Ideally the back is straight, perpendicular to the ground. You may interlace the fingers with the arms on the floor, pointing away from the body. Continue Breath of Fire for **1 to 2 mintues**. As you breath, slowly and carefully stretch the legs farther away from the torso so that you feel a mild stretch in the upper back and neck. Then inhale deeply. Exhale and relax the breath. Slowly come out of the posture by releasing the spine, vertebra by vertebra, from the top of the spine to its base. Then relax on the back.

These exercises open the upper spine and related nerve passages to the flow of Kundalini energy. They also stimulate the thyroid and parathyroid glands.

8. **Sat Kriya in Celibate Pose**. Sit on the heels in Rock Pose. Spread the knees and heels wide so that you are sitting between the heels in **Celibate Pose**. Clasp the hands above the head in Venus Lock, fingers interlaced except for the index fingers, which point straight up. (Men cross the right thumb over the left; women cross left thumb over right.) Arms are straight, hugging the ears. Squeeze the Navel Point in and up as you say S*at*. Release as you chant *Naam*. Continue for **3 to 5 minutes**. To end, inhale and squeeze the muscles tightly from the buttocks all the way up the back. Mentally allow the energy to flow through the top of the skull. Exhale and relax.

This exercise circulates the Kundalini and integrates the energy released from the lower three chakras into the entire system so that the total effects of these exercises are stable and long lasting. (See page 10 for more detailed description of Sat Kriya.)

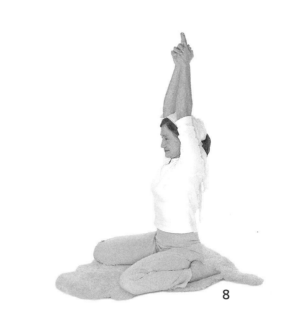

8

9. **Deep Relaxation**. Deeply relax for **3 to 10 minutes**.

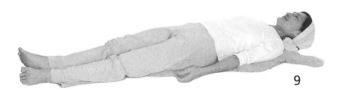

9

About This Kriya

As human beings, we share certain instincts with animals, but we also have the ability to direct, shape and give meaning to the expression of these instincts. Many of the strongest instincts find expression and representation through the Lower Triangle of chakras, which include the First, Second and Third Chakras. The physical correlates of these chakras are the rectum, the sex organs and the Navel Point.

Dysfunctions of the body are reflected in the mind and vice versa. A serious neurotic behavior or self-destructive attitude will also appear as an imbalance in the Lower Triangle. One of the most direct ways to correct such an imbalance is to physically stimulate the nervous and glandular systems in order to alter the instinctual and learned patterns in the lower chakras. Once this is achieved and a new energy balance is attained, then, through analytic self-assessment and meditation, it is possible to effect the wholistic change in behavior which is desired.

This kriya is an example of such a technology. To use it correctly, remember to focus the mind on what you are doing and experiencing during this kriya.

KRIYA FOR A **CALM & OPEN HEART**

JANUARY 24, 1990

1. Sit in Easy Pose with a straight spine and stretch the tongue out. Breathe in and out powerfully and deeply through the mouth. Open up the lungs. **2 minutes**.

2. Using the tip of the tongue moving rapidly against the upper palate, make the sound *"la, la, la, la."* It is like a continuous, high-pitched warble. **2 minutes**.
Making this sound stimulates the brow area, and will relax you. In the Middle East, women use this sound to send their men off to battle and to welcome them home.

3. Touch the thumb to the mound under the Mercury finger and close the fist around it. With the palms facing down, rapidly revolve the fists around each other in outward circles. Keep the revolving fists in front of your Heart Center. **2 minutes**.
This is a very fast movement and is beneficial for the heart.

4. Extend the arms straight in front, parallel to the floor, with the palms facing each other. Keep the elbows straight and move each arm alternately up and down approximately one to two feet. **1 minute**.
This motion will adjust the rib cage.

5. Extend the arms straight in front at a 60 degree angle. The palms are facing down. There is no bend in the elbows. Rapidly open and close the hands so that the fingers slap the palms, creating a magnetic shock. **2 minutes**.
This exercise invigorates the brain.

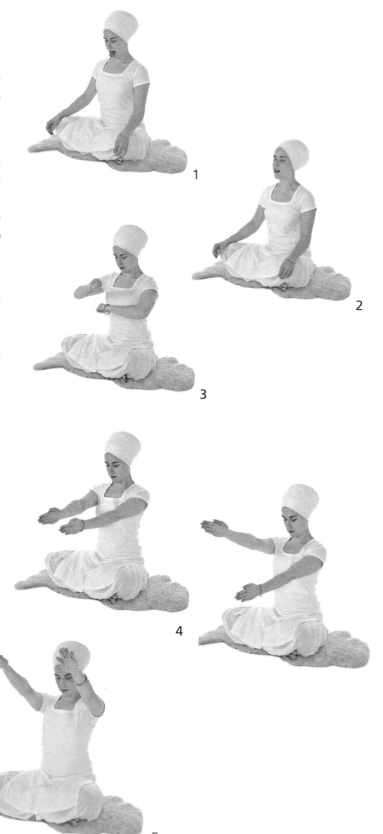

6. **Sufi Grind**. Sitting in Easy Pose with the hands on the knees, rotate the torso in a counter-clockwise motion. Grind the spine firmly and powerfully. **2 minutes.**

7. **Body Drops**. Support yourself with the hands on either side of the hips. Lift the hips off the floor and let them drop back down. Move very quickly. Your entire weight will be supported by your hands. **1 1/2 minutes.**

8. Interlock the fingers behind the neck. Keep the spine straight and focus at the tip of the nose. Meditate to Nirinjan Kaur's recording of *Rakhe Rakhan Har*, listening to the beat of your Heart Center. **7 minutes.**

9. Remain in the posture and keep eyes focused at the tip of the nose. Forcefully pump the navel to the beat of Guru Shabad Singh's recording of *Pavan Pavan* for **13 Minutes.** *This exercise gives you mastery over the Pranic Shakti, the life force energy, by using the navel to develop stamina and inner strength.*

TO END: Inhale, suspend the breath for 10 seconds and exhale. Repeat this sequence two more times and relax. Raise the hands overhead and shake them.

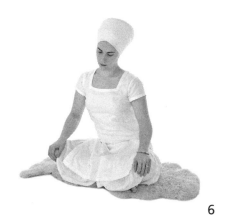

6

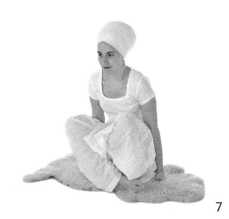

7

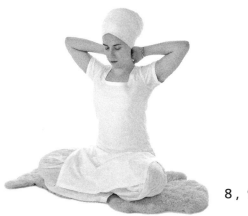

8 , 9

About This Kriya
"As long as the mind is dark and does not let the light of the soul shine in your life, you will never have the joy and success that is your birthright as a human." — Yogi Bhajan

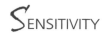

BEAMING AND **CREATING THE FUTURE**

JUNE 12, 1990

POSTURE: Sit in Easy Pose. Stretch the spine up and become very still.

EYE FOCUS: Eyes are closed.

MUDRA: Relax the hands in Gyan Mudra across the knees.

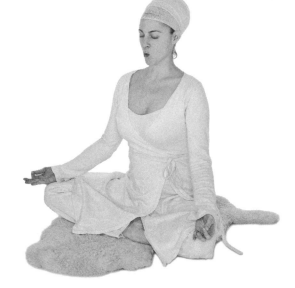

PART ONE
Drink the breath in a single, deep, long sip through a rounded mouth. Close the mouth and exhale through the nose, slowly and completely. **7-15 minutes.**

PART TWO
Inhale and hold the breath comfortably. As you suspend the breath in, meditate on zero. Think in this way: *"All is zero; I am zero; each thought is zero; my pain is zero; that problem is zero; that illness is zero."* Meditate on all negative, emotional, mental and physical conditions and situations. As each thing crosses the mind, bring it to zero—a single point of light, a small, insignificant non-existence. Exhale and repeat. Breathe in a comfortable rhythm. **7-11 minutes.**

PART THREE
Think of the quality or condition you most desire for your complete happiness and growth. Summarize it in a single word like *"Wealth," "Health," "Relationship," "Guidance," "Knowledge," "Luck."* It has to be one word. Lock on that word and thought. Visualize facets of it. Inhale and suspend the breath as you beam the thought in a continuous stream. Lock onto it. Relax the breath as needed. **5-15 minutes.**

TO END: Inhale and move the shoulders, arms and spine. Then stretch the arms up, spread the fingers wide, and breathe deeply a few times.

About This Meditation

After clearing the mind of other distracting thoughts and attachments, it has tremendous capacity and creativity when focused and beaming. Use that beaming faculty. Become still and project the mind to create your future and your relationship to the world. The best way to practice this is on an empty stomach with only liquids taken during the day.

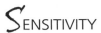

MEDITATION TO **REMEMBER THE HEAVENS**

JULY 2, 1998

POSTURE: Sit in Easy Pose with a straight spine, and a light Neck Lock.

MUDRA: Stretch the right arm out in front at a 60 degree angle. Palm is flat and face down, fingers and thumbs straight. Hold the position. Bend the left elbow into the left side, flat palm facing straight forward, fingers straight, pointing towards the ceiling. The center of the palm of the hand is held at shoulder height. Stretch the shoulders back a bit.

EYE FOCUS: Eyes are closed.

BREATH: Make the mouth into a firm "O" and inhale as if you are drinking water through the mouth. Exhale through the nose.
This hiss can take all the poisons from the body.

TIME: 16 1/2 minutes.

TO END: Inhale deeply, tighten the left hand, tighten and stretch the right arm up. Create a balance in the body, and give strength to the spine. Hold **10-25 seconds**. Exhale. Inhale a second time, stretch and hold **5-15 seconds**. Exhale. Inhale a third time, repeat, hold **5-15 seconds**. Relax.

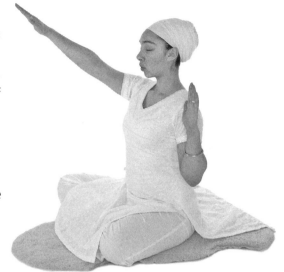

About This Meditation

It is the central nervous system within the spine which you are challenging with this meditation.

"Don't let yourself down, don't let anybody down, and do not participate in any letdown or gossip, if you want to practice gospel. Understand that. These few things are there for you to know. You cannot live on this Earth without respect and reverence. Do not value life by gain and loss of the Earth. Value life with gain and loss of the Heavens and Mother Earth. The majority of you forget the Heavens and that's not what we need." — Yogi Bhajan

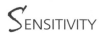

MERCURY PROJECTION MEDITATION

OCTOBER 1996

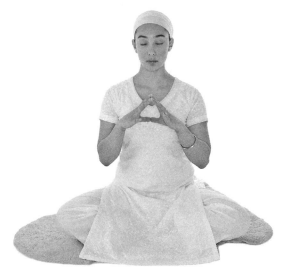

POSTURE: Sit in Easy Pose with a straight spine, and a light Neck Lock.

MUDRA & MOVEMENT: Elbows are bent at the sides. Place the hands in front of the Heart Center, palms facing each other, fingers pointing straight up, and spread slightly apart. Stretch the thumbs back, pointing towards the chest. Bring the tips of the thumbs, index & middle fingers together. They will form a sort of triangle.

The ring and pinkie fingers do not touch, and are separated from one another by several inches. The palms are also stretched wide apart.

Holding the mudra, bring the palms toward one another slightly, just until the tips of the pinkie fingers can touch. Note: Make sure that the ring fingertips do NOT touch.

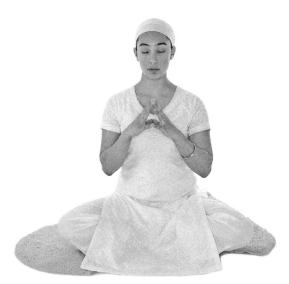

MANTRA: Chant the mantra *Wahe Guru* in a continuous monotone, with a steady rhythm. Repeat the mantra one full time in position (a), and then chant the mantra one full time in position (b). Continue. Each repetition takes about 1 1/2 seconds. Pronounce each syllable distinctly:

> *WHAA - HAY GU-ROO*

EYE FOCUS: Focus is at the tip of the nose.

TIME: 3-11 minutes.

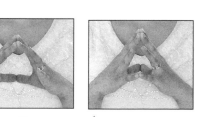

About This Meditation

"This is called the 'Mercury Projection.' Mercury is the Lord of Communication, the Star of Communication. This meditation will make your mind most alert. You as a human cannot afford to be wrong. You want to be a yogi? I think all these mudras and postures are meant to put in us infinite alertness. Sometimes the rhythmic flare of the Sun differs with the magnetic rhythm of the under flow of the Earth. Technically this meditation is for the control of the Mercury influence in you. The little finger is connected to Mercury." — Yogi Bhajan

THE SONG OF VICTORY

I-AANRHEE-AY MAANRA KAA-E KARAY-EH

JANUARY 6, 1980

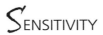

Shabd Guru

"Try to understand this shabd. It is one of the secrets to every woman's happiness. This is the Guru's Message in this shabd: Why are you looking outside yourself? What are you looking for? For glory, for domestic life, for nothing? What are you looking for? Appreciation? From the people who tell you to have white skin, the people who tell you that you are great? What people tell you means nothing if, in your own consciousness, you don't recognize your greatness. What people say doesn't matter. This is why people in America are freaking out and falling apart, because they want people to tell them, "You are great." I tell you: outside bait will never make you great. It is your own internal voice that has to tell you that you are great—and it is that greatness, which is Godliness. Stop seeking outside for the nectar. There is nothing to find outside, if the inside is hollow and empty. That's the meaning of this shabd. Take it to heart."

—Yogi Bhajan

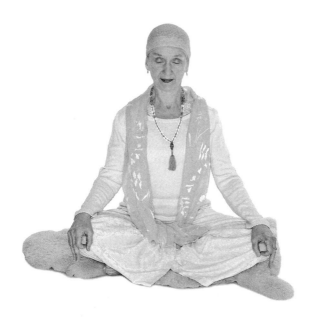

ਵਿਆਨੜੀਏ ਮਾਨੜਾ ਕਾਇ ਕਰੇਹਿ

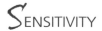
THE SONG OF VICTORY
I-AANRHEE-AY MAANRA KAA-E KARAY-EH

Guru Nanak, Siri Guru Granth Sahib page 722

ਤਿਲੰਗ ਮਃ੧

ਇਆਨੜੀਏ ਮਾਨੜਾ ਕਾਇ ਕਰੇਹਿ

ਆਪਨੜੈ ਘਰਿ ਹਰਿ ਰੰਗੋ ਕੀ ਨ ਮਾਣੇਹਿ

ਸਹੁ ਨੇੜੈ ਧਨ ਕੰਮਲੀਏ ਬਾਹਰੁ ਕਿਆ ਢੂਢੇਹਿ

ਭੈ ਕੀਆ ਦੇਹਿ ਸਲਾਈਆ ਨੈਨੀ ਭਾਵ ਕਾ ਕਰਿ ਸੀਗਾਰੋ

ਤਾ ਸੋਹਾਗਣਿ ਜਾਣੀਐ ਲਾਗੀ ਜਾ ਸਹੁ ਧਰੇ ਪਿਆਰੋ ॥੧॥

ਇਆਣੀ ਬਾਲੀ ਕਿਆ ਕਰੇ ਜਾ ਧਨ ਕੰਤ ਨ ਭਾਵੈ

ਕਰਣ ਪਲਾਹ ਕਰੇ ਬਹੁਤੇਰੇ ਸਾ ਧਨ ਮਹਲੁ ਨ ਪਾਵੈ

ਵਿਣੁ ਕਰਮਾ ਕਿਛੁ ਪਾਈਐ ਨਾਹੀ ਜੇ ਬਹੁਤੇਰਾ ਧਾਵੈ

ਲਬ ਲੋਭ ਅਹੰਕਾਰ ਕੀ ਮਾਤੀ ਮਾਇਆ ਮਾਹਿ ਸਮਾਣੀ

ਇਨੀ ਬਾਤੀ ਸਹੁ ਪਾਈਐ ਨਾਹੀ ਭਈ ਕਾਮਣਿ ਇਆਣੀ ॥੨॥

ਜਾਇ ਪੁਛਹੁ ਸੋਹਾਗਣੀ ਵਾਹੈ ਕਿਨੀ ਬਾਤੀ ਸਹੁ ਪਾਈਐ

ਜੋ ਕਿਛੁ ਕਰੇ ਸੋ ਭਲਾ ਕਰਿ ਮਾਨੀਐ ਹਿਕਮਤਿ ਹੁਕਮੁ ਚੁਕਾਈਐ

ਜਾ ਕੈ ਪ੍ਰੇਮਿ ਪਦਾਰਥੁ ਪਾਈਐ ਤਉ ਚਰਣੀ ਚਿਤੁ ਲਾਈਐ

ਸਹੁ ਕਹੈ ਸੋ ਕੀਜੈ ਤਨੁ ਮਨੋ ਦੀਜੈ ਐਸਾ ਪਰਮਲੁ ਲਾਈਐ

ਏਵ ਕਹਹਿ ਸੋਹਾਗਣੀ ਭੈਨੇ ਇਨੀ ਬਾਤੀ ਸਹੁ ਪਾਈਐ ॥੩॥

ਆਪੁ ਗਵਾਈਐ ਤਾ ਸਹੁ ਪਾਈਐ ਅਉਰੁ ਕੈਸੀ ਚਤੁਰਾਈ

ਸਹੁ ਨਦਰਿ ਕਰਿ ਦੇਖੈ ਸੋ ਦਿਨੁ ਲੇਖੈ ਕਾਮਣਿ ਨਉ ਨਿਧਿ ਪਾਈ

ਆਪਣੇ ਕੰਤ ਪਿਆਰੀ ਸਾ ਸੋਹਾਗਣਿ ਨਾਨਕ ਸਾ ਸਭਰਾਈ

ਐਸੇ ਰੰਗਿ ਰਾਤੀ ਸਹਜ ਕੀ ਮਾਤੀ ਅਹਿਨਿਸਿ ਭਾਇ ਸਮਾਣੀ

ਸੁੰਦਰਿ ਸਾਇ ਸਰੂਪ ਬਿਚਖਣਿ ਕਹੀਐ ਸਾ ਸਿਆਣੀ ॥੪॥੨॥੪॥

TILANG, FIRST MEHL

I-aanrhee-ay maanrhaa kaa-ay karayhi.
apnarhai ghar har rango kee na maaneh.
Saho nayrhai dhan kammlee-ay baahar ki-aa dhoodhayhi.
Bhai kee-aa deh salaa-ee-aa nainee bhaav kaa kar seegaaro.
Taa sohagan jaanee-ai laagee jaa saho dharay pi-aaro.   1

I-aanee baalee ki-aa karay jaa dhan kant na bhaavai.
Karan palaah karay bahutayray saa dhan mahal na paavai.
Vin karmaa kichh paa-ee-ai naahee jay bahutayraa dhaavai.
Lab lobh ahaNkaar kee maatee maa-i-aa maahi samaanee.
Inee baatee saho paa-ee-ai naahee bha-ee kaaman i-aanee. 2

Jaa-ay puchhahu sohaaganee vaahai kinee baatee saho paa-ee-ai.
Jo kichh karay so bhalaa kar maaneeai hikmat hukam chukhaa-ee-ai
Jaa kai paraym padaarath paa-eeai ta-o charnee chit laa-ee-ai.
Saho kahai so keejai tan mano deejai aisaa parmal laa-ee-ai.
Ayv kaheh sohaaganee bhainay inee baatee saho paa-ee-ai.   3

Aap gavaa-ee-ai taa saho paa-ee-ai a-or kaisee chaturaa-ee.
Saho nadar kar daykhai so din laykhai kaaman na-o niDh paa-ee.
Aapnay kant pi-aaree saa sohagan naanak saa sabhraa-ee.
Aisay rang raatee sahj kee maatee ahinis bhaa-ay samaanee.
sundar saa-ay saroop bichkhan kahee-ai saa si-aanee.   4/2/4

RAAG TILANG FIRST CHANNEL OF LIGHT GURU NANAK

Oh, innocent woman, what can that one to whom you look with reverence do?
In his own House he does not look to, does not listen to, this graceful one, his beloved one.
He is so near to you, so attached to you, what is he trying to find outside. Where is the discrepancy in the relationship?
Put in your eyes the realization, the charisma of fear and go deeply, telescopically, into his being to find
what you have been missing in his personality. Then decorate yourself with reverence for him;
by your glow and radiance you will yourself receive reverence. Then only are you married,
at that level of consciousness, one with Him, so that you can seat Him in your heart with love.
What can this innocent woman do if she cannot reach to His Essence?
There must be something hidden in His character, approach, language, behavior, or the environments.
She may do everything, often she overdoes it, but does not get to the core of His being.
Unless that happens your relationship will not prosper.

—Translation by Yogi Bhajan

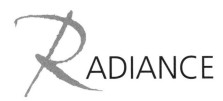ADIANCE

WALKING IN BEAUTY & LIVING BY GRACE

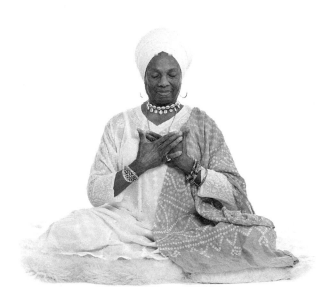

THE QUALITIES OF CONTENTMENT, serenity, and containment build the strength of our Arclines, which give us an indescribably beautiful radiance and guide us to victory. It is our time as women to stand tall, walk in our beauty, live in our grace and be the divine leaders of the Aquarian Age and the generations to follow.

THERE WAS A TIME WHEN WOMAN WAS WORSHIPPED for her divinity, her beauty, her wisdom and her grace. In the eyes of the newborn infant and their perfect innocence, looking into the eyes of the Mother, this has never changed. The child sees not just the physical form of the mother but the light or radiance that surrounds and emanates from her physical body. This is the image of woman that Yogi Bhajan saw and nurtured within us.

Many of us have spent years basing our self-worth on whether we met the standards that media and culture have set for women: to be skinny and sexy in order to be truly a woman. How liberating it is to think of our value being defined by our inner light, our radiance and grace.

Each of us is unique and as women we have been given a gift, the beguiling beauty of God within us. Yogi Bhajan said if God ever thought of taking only one form, woman would be the vehicle in which God would come to Earth. Our beauty is not in our makeup or our fashion, it lies in our depth.

The strength of our mental, spiritual, auric, subtle, pranic and radiant bodies forms a brilliant light field—our radiance—and makes up our entire physical being. Add to that radiance our smile and nothing can defeat us. With this strength and contentment there is no need for trauma and drama because your attraction will be so strong that everything will come to you.

We have another blessing as women that gives us effectiveness and radiance—our grace. What is grace? Grace is the strength of character to be you and to never let yourself down or anyone else down. Woman walking in her radiance and grace requires no introduction. We do not have to

utter a word to be noticed or for people to show us the reverence, trust and understanding we deserve. Woman with her one smile can heal and transform all that surrounds her. Our power and strength come from manifesting who we truly are. *I am a woman, I am a graceful woman.* When we hold this consciousness, we excel.

Our challenge as women is not to be defined by the standards of outer beauty that our culture demands of us, but instead to live in contentment, serenity and containment. These qualities build the strength of our Arclines, which give us an indescribably beautiful radiance and guide us to victory. It is our time as women to stand tall, walk in our beauty, live in our grace and be the divine leaders of the Aquarian Age and the generations to follow.

EACH OF THE KRIYAS AND MEDITATIONS in this section bring great vitality and radiance to the physical and radiant bodies. Negativity is eliminated, and loneliness and depression are rooted out on a deep cellular level. The set to make you Enchantingly Beautiful gives a glow to your skin and a radiance in your face. To understand, in the depth of your being, and recite the *shabd, Bhand Jamee-ai,* will give you the knowledge of what it means to be a woman and to live in your grace and divinity. Beauty is within. May your radiance glow like a sun and may all who see you be healed and uplifted by your presence.

PRITPAL KAUR KHALSA
ESPAÑOLA, NEW MEXICO

KRIYA TO MAKE YOU ENCHANTINGLY BEAUTIFUL

1. **Spine Flex Variation**. Sit on the heels in Rock Pose. Put the palms flat on the ground outside of the knees, a little to the front. Pull the neck up, spine straight. You should look just like one of those little Buddhist temple lions. Begin flexing the spine to its maximum capacity, keeping the elbows straight. Inhale, flex forward, exhale powerfully, flex backward. Keep a steady rhythm. The forehead will get hot and the spine will sweat. Continue for **3 minutes**. *This exercise purifies the blood, adds strength to the whole nervous system and will save you from back and shoulder pain.*
Move immediately into the next exercise.

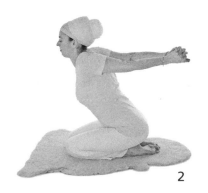

2. **Yoga Mudra**. Still in Rock Pose, interlace the fingers at the base of the spine with palms facing the head. Straighten the arms and lift as high as you can. **2 minutes**. Inhale, exhale, relax.
This exercise puts such circulation and beauty into your cheeks that you will not need cosmetics.

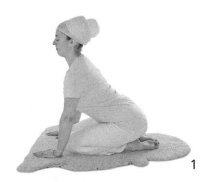

3. Sit with the legs straight in front, heels together. Place the palms down at the sides of the body, slightly in back of the hips. Raise the legs slowly to 60 degrees and hold. Don't bend backward at all. **3 minutes**. Inhale and exhale 2 times.
This exercise stretches the sciatic nerve and helps relieve headaches.

Move immediately into the next exercise.

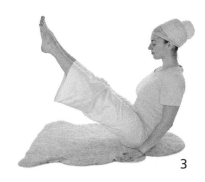

4. With the body in the same position as #3, bring the knees onto the chest. Balance the body, holding the feet 6" off the ground. Begin Breath of Fire for **2 minutes**. Inhale, exhale, relax.
This exercise cleans the blood with 50 powerful repetitions of Breath of Fire. As long as the breath is continuous, it cleans the lungs and stimulates the life force so that you can retain your youth and power.

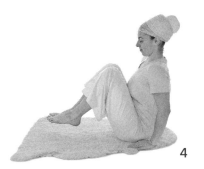

5. Stretch the legs straight in front and catch the toes. Elbows are straight. Pull and elongate the spine fully, and pull Neck Lock. Close the eyes, and roll them up. Press the toes hard. **2 minutes**.

6. Maintain the same position as Exercise 5, and begin to chant the mantra **HUM**. It means **WE**. The sound is continuous. *This helps you come out of individual pettiness and tension. It cleans the lungs and creates such a stimulation to the life force that you can retain your youth, power, and potency.*
Exercises 5 and 6 stimulate the two master glands of the blood— the liver and the spleen. If you stretch very tight and concentrate as you keep up, you may see colors and other visual effects. It is only an experience, so press beyond this point.

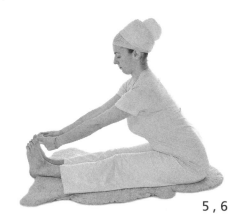

5 , 6

About This Kriya

The purpose of this set is to make you enchantingly beautiful. This short kriya can make you a different person. It increases your beauty, physically and mentally. Many of us have lost contact with the essence of beauty, which comes from good physical condition. It is a radiance of soul that shines through the physical appearance and beyond. This series elevates you to a level of consciousness where you can appreciate the new inflow of energy. It makes you want to meditate.

KEEPING THE **BODY BEAUTIFUL**
OCTOBER 1969

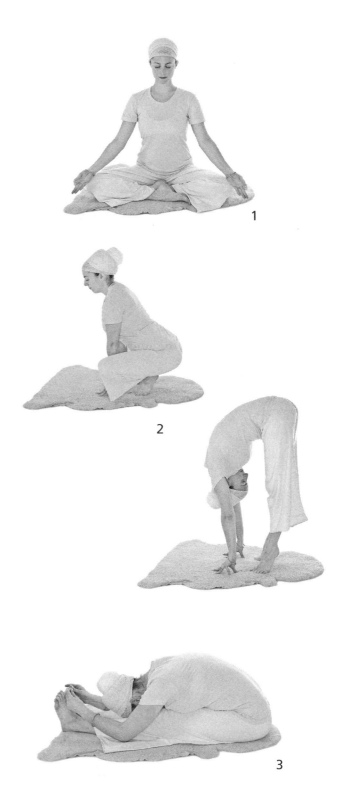

1. **Long Deep Breathing**. Sit in Easy Pose with spine straight. Begin breathing long and deep through both nostrils. Focus on the life-giving flow of breath for **3 minutes**. To end, inhale, suspend the breath a few seconds, then relax the breath.

2. **Frog Pose**. Squat down on the toes, knees wide apart. Heels are touching, and raised up off the ground. Place the fingertips on the ground between the knees. The face is forward. Inhale as you raise the hips up (2a), keeping the fingertips on the ground, heels up, knees locked.

Exhale down (2b), face forward, knees outside of arms. **10 times**. On the tenth, stay down and take three deep breaths. On the third breath exhale completely and suspend the breath out as you apply *mulbandh*. Suspend the breath out 10-20 seconds.

Repeat **Frog Pose 26 times**. On the last time, stay down and take three deep breaths. On the third breath, suspend the breath out and again apply *mulbandh*. *Feel energy rise along the spine as you suspend the breath out. Do not strain.*

3. **Front Stretch**. Stretch the legs out straight in front. Relax forward and grab the big toes in Finger Lock (Index finger and middle finger pull the toe, and the thumb presses on the toe.) Inhale, lengthening the spine. Exhale, bend forward from the navel, bringing chest to thighs, nose to knees. The head follows last. Avoid leading with the head. Hold the position for **3 minutes**.

continued next page

About This Kriya

This kriya, which contains a slight variation of the standard Frog Pose, is very powerful. You must keep the chin locked in. It readjusts the sex energy and the balance of *prana* and *apana*. It is good for digestion and brings circulation to the head. If done with powerful breaths it will make you sweat quickly.

The body is a temple of human expression and evolvement. We are often told by the media and friends that it wears out, has many illnesses, and is extremely fragile. In fact, the body is sensitive and self-repairing. As Yogi Bhajan puts it:

"This beautiful body cannot be eaten by anything except your own ego. God doesn't kill you. There is no death except your own ego, and your own negativity, which reduces the voltage of your life force so your circumvent field becomes weak and death creeps into your body. This body is beautiful. It was made by a very special imagination of the Creator.

People search for the experience of God, the experience of freedom, energy, and consciousness. If we would only purify ourselves, then God would be known to us and come to live in us. That infinite energy is the giver in every situation. We recognize it by cleaning, caring, and utilizing what we have already been given."

Our own habits of possession, constriction, anger, tension, and attachment set up energy patterns within the body that disrupt the normal flow of vital energy. This opens the door to disease, both physical and mental. After all, we are creators also, and, to a certain extent, create the environments we want to live in. We create our bodies with each thought and activity, as well as with each meal. So we need to clean the body and readjust the flow of energy periodically since we are all products of our habits and since few of us are without ego.

OLD GYPSY WAY OF CALLING ON THE SPIRIT

JULY 4, 1994

POSTURE: Sit in Easy Pose with a straight spine, and a light Neck Lock.

MUDRA: Raise the arms up 60 degrees from horizontal, elbows and wrists straight. Stretch the body forward slightly from the plane of the body. The angle of the palms follows the angle of the arms. The fingers are straight and together, thumbs relaxed.

VISUALIZATION: Imagine a flame at the Heart Center. Do not move.

BREATH: Breathe consciously, long and deep.

TIME: 3 minutes.

TO END: Inhale deeply with a prayer for the loftiness of Creator Mother Earth and peace. Hold for 15 seconds. Exhale. Inhale deeply. Feel in your heart the blessing of the Divine Mother. Hold for 15 seconds. Exhale. Inhale deep. Feel the taste of the sweetness of life. Hold for 15 seconds. Exhale.

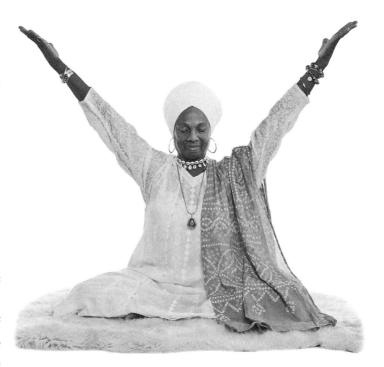

About This Meditation

Invoke the spirit of Mother Earth with your own body. Feel the flame bright and powerful at the intersection of a line from nipple to nipple, and a line from nose to navel.

MEDITATION TO DEVELOP THE RADIANT BODY
JULY 31, 2001

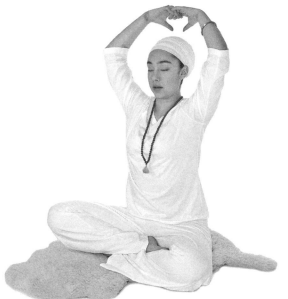

POSTURE: Sit in Easy Pose with a straight spine, and a light Neck Lock.

MUDRA: Arc the arms over the head, with the fingers interlocked in-between the palms. Tuck the chin in, and pull the arms back and slightly downward until the hands are above the back of the neck.

MANTRA: Chant the *Ik Acharee Chand shabd*:

Ajai Alai Abhai Abai
Abhoo Ajoo Anaas Akaas
Aganj Abhanj Alakh Abhakh
Akaal Dyaal Alaykh Abhaykh
Anaam Akaam Agaahaa Adhaahaa
Anaathay Pramaathay Ajonee Amonee
Na Raagay Na Rangay Na Roopay Na Raykay
Akaramang Abharamang Aganjay Alaykhay

(Recording by Gurushabd Singh and Nirinjan Kaur recommended.)

TIME: 11-22 minutes.

TO END: Inhale deeply, suspend the breath and stretch the arms up high keeping the fingers interlaced. Exhale powerfully. Repeat 2 more times. Relax, shake out the hands

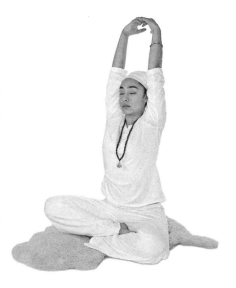

About This Kriya

This extraordinary meditation is to be done with great precision. Make sure the hand mudra and the position of the hands over the head are held correctly and fixed.

As you do the *Ik Acharee Chand* mantra of Guru Gobind Singh, hear each word as a world—each word as complete as you speak, projecting with the Fifth Chakra and vibrating the sound as *naad* with the Eighth Chakra.

This will build and expand the Radiant Body. It is through this expanded Radiant Body that we can hold the link and space as teachers. With that radiance our communication becomes impersonally personal. It is natural to give gratitude to the Golden Link, to our teacher Yogi Bhajan and to show reverence for the sacred space of the teacher within and without.

When the Radiant Body is depleted, we feel we have to do everything. We're better than some people and worse than others. When your hidden agendas are put aside and your radiance is strong, your presence embodies your teacher. You are beyond comparison and act in love and duty to your students. You teach in the name of the teacher and take no finite claim. You act in love and dissolve yourself in the rhythms of infinity without hesitation. Without the full Radiant Body we grasp for some security other than our Being and the Infinite. With the Radiant Body strong, our presence communicates contentment, containment, completeness and consciousness.

EVENING MEDITATION AGAINST LONELINESS AND RESTLESSNESS
SHABD SHU GADHARA KRIYA WITH KARAM SHAMBAVI MUDRA
MAY 2, 1972

PART ONE
POSTURE: Sit in Easy Pose with a straight spine, and a light Neck Lock.

MUDRA: Elbows are relaxed down by the sides, the forearms are in line with the thighs, palms up, parallel to the ground. Fingers are in receptive Gyan Mudra.

EYE FOCUS: Focus is at the Third Eye Point. Feel it as the apex of a triangle with the hands.

MANTRA: Inhale in 4 strokes mentally vibrating:

> *SAT SAT SAT SAT*

Exhale in one long stroke mentally vibrating:

> *NAAM*

TIME: Continue for **11 minutes**. (Build up to 31 minutes over time.)

TO END: Inhale and tip the head back. Then bring the head level.

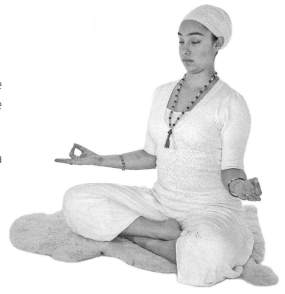
PART ONE

PART TWO
Sit on the left heel, right leg stretched out in front. Grasp the big toe of the outstretched foot with the right hand. Pulling back on the toe, grab the heel of the same foot with the left hand. Breath automatically as you chant:

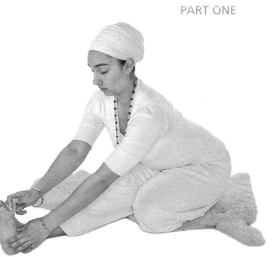
PART TWO

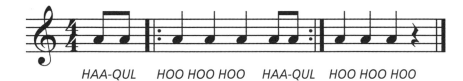

HAA-QUL   HOO HOO HOO   HAA-QUL   HOO HOO HOO

TIME: Not specified. Suggest **3 minutes**.

PART THREE

Sit in Easy Pose or Lotus Pose. Place the arms between the legs, hands under the buttocks. Let the head fall back, point the chin up. Mentally concentrate from the rectum to the chin. Inhale in **4 strokes** mentally vibrating:

SAT SAT SAT SAT

Exhale in one long breath mentally vibrating:

NAAM

TIME: Continue for **11 minutes**. (Build to 31 minutes with time.)

TO END: Inhale and bring the neck straight. Folllow immediately with deep relaxation.

DEEP RELAXATION: It is important to follow with **11 minutes** of relaxation.

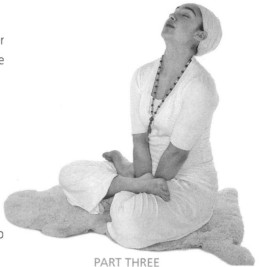

PART THREE

About This Meditation

The first two parts of this kriya create an active seal of consciousness to bring triple changes: in the physical, in the mental, and in the totality of the being, working on the positive ego. Part Three addresses the negative ego, and can bring unruly thoughts, so must be practiced with Part One and Part Two, and followed by a deep relaxation. If you become irritated when you begin practicing this kriya, add the practice of the kriya: Movement Relaxation. (Movement Relaxation Series is on page 173.)

This kriya balances the ego, conquers the fear of death, promotes sound sleep, eliminates strange dreams, and gives a positive attitude. It produces a vitality in the etheric body so that it becomes extremely strong and totally regulates the glands. Thus the emotions become constant and the mind becomes divine.

This kriya is traditionally called: Shabd Shu Gadhara Kriya (Karam Shambavi Mudra) and is to be done at the two weak points of the day, when negativity may triumph. This is when the the sun is at 60 degrees: approximately 3 hours after sunrise, and at sunset. This is especially helpful in the evening, when you can become lonely and restless. All negative acts start in the evening. This kriya eliminates negativity. You will not be betrayed in life or love if you meditate on Infinity in the evening when Venus comes up.

In life there are constant waves of emotions, yet life is not these waves. The highest point of consciousness in life is love, but love is a constant frequency of vibrations throughout life which has no condition in it. The problem with us is that the positive and negative aspects of the ego are not balanced, so no neutrality and consistency can take root. Positive ego is the constant vibratory projection of the self. Negative ego is the over-projection or under-contraction of the self. The imbalance of these two makes us unable to conquer the fear of death, so we resist changing and evolving to higher consciousness, since every real change is experienced as a death.

"How can your Creator and Mother Nature who created you allow you to be lonely? There are beautiful trees, beautiful times; everywhere around you beauty is in such abundance that if you look ahead, you can enjoy and enjoy, forever and ever. Why do you feel lonely? Why do you want to be recognized? Why do you overextend yourself and make yourself weak?

This is how you distribute your time: You give 60-70% to your ego; 40% to your imaginations; 10-15% to self-pity. So, you give about 40-60% to your insecurities. At best, you give from 3-5% of your time to your own divinity. A person who gives 10-15% of his time to his divinity is considered a saint.

Give your evenings to happiness on Earth, and your mornings to God. If you watch TV at night, you can't get up, it takes away all your energy. Evening is a time of peace and rest. Make sure evenings are passed in elevated human relationship. Avoid any situation which will drag you down. Be in the company of the holy." —Yogi Bhajan

WOMAN'S IDENTITY

BHAND JAMEE-AI

JULY 23, 1984

Shabd Guru

"I want to speak literally. You are in command and within the flow. What do we mean by command? That is a very accurate question. Let us see what the dictionary says. I know what I mean, but what the dictionary tells us will be good for all of us to know, too. Bring the dictionary and find the word "command." Some people think command means control, which every woman likes to feel.

"From the dictionary: Command—to order, to exercise authority over, to rule, to dominate by location (Yogi Bhajan comments, "Location, mind you, means space"); the act of giving orders, an order so given, the authority to give them, ability to control, mastery, a leader or person under the control of one officer.

"You are in the command of the flow. What is the flow? Every breath is the flow of life. You must command it. Whether you want to retreat, hold the breath, extend the breath, move the breath, whatever your life is, you should be in command, not the environment or circumstances; not the games and not the loss. Is that clear? My expertise is that I try to make people feel the 'You' within their 'you'. It is my experience that once a woman finds her Self within herself, she is out of the woods, free from any and all danger. That's what I have been trying to do for the past eight years. Nothing is lost if you do not lose this chance. A woman who is not one step ahead of a man and a man who is not one step ahead of the time are failures. Try your best.

"A woman must be in the now and be 18 hours ahead, too. Man cannot be ahead more than 12 hours normally, so you just figure out 18 hours ahead—and understand the now—and you will be loved, kissed and hugged so much you won't believe it. They love it—that kind of woman is very juicy to a man. A woman who knows the art of how not to break communication, how not to push the point and bring about anger, and who can figure out 18-20 hours ahead of a man yet always keep her consciousness and her senses in the now, is a queen. Nobody can take away her majesty. Just remember these few things.

"The greatest weapon with which you can win is to prove you are reliable. Once you can establish with a man that you are reliable, you have him forever. It doesn't matter how nasty, down-to-earth and perverted or inverted that man may be. Don't misunderstand at all. Once a woman becomes a woman, man has no defense at all; because the woman contains the man, just as the spider contains the web within it.

"Look, woman. Life is for you! It's easy! It is all for you. Look at the world of the man. He marries a woman. He runs after a woman. He beats a woman. He squanders a woman. He loves a woman. He goes against woman. If you look at all this, it's just nonsense; it doesn't make any sense. It all revolves around a woman. That's why Guru Nanak could sing so openly:

Bhand jamee-ai bhand nimee-ai bhand mangan vee-aaho.
In a woman we are conceived, and from a woman we are born. With a woman, man is betrothed and married.

"This is every man's character. Every woman should know this shabd. Every woman should know what a man is. In this one *shabd*, Guru Nanak has totally explained what life is about. It's so well explained. There's no second thought needed. If you keep that one shabd in your memory, you can always know what this whole world is about. No greater attribute can be paid to a woman than that one line: *Bhaagaa ratee chaar.* She is the exclusive master of fortune in the fourth domain of all ethers, in essence, in quality, in projection and in depth. This one phrase has that kind of meaning: "In all four channels of essence of the planetary virtue, magnetic and subtle, she is the domain." And it can go on and on, beautiful words, *bhaagaa ratee chaar.* That is the woman of my imagination, about whom Guru Nanak sang.

"What is the last line? *Jit mukh sadaa saalaahe-ai bhaagaa ratee chaar.* Translate it and then you will find out how virtuous, how bountiful, how beautiful, how wonderful, how graceful, how full of everything you are as a woman."

—Yogi Bhajan

WOMAN'S IDENTITY
BHAND JAMEE-AI

Guru Nanak, Siri Guru Granth Sahib page 473

ਮਃ 1

ਭੰਡਿ ਜੰਮੀਐ ਭੰਡਿ ਨਿੰਮੀਐ ਭੰਡਿ ਮੰਗਣੁ ਵੀਆਹੁ

ਭੰਡਹੁ ਹੋਵੈ ਦੋਸਤੀ ਭੰਡਹੁ ਚਲੈ ਰਾਹੁ

ਭੰਡੁ ਮੂਆ ਭੰਡੁ ਭਾਲੀਐ ਭੰਡਿ ਹੋਵੈ ਬੰਧਾਨੁ

ਸੋ ਕਿਉ ਮੰਦਾ ਆਖੀਐ ਜਿਤੁ ਜੰਮਹਿ ਰਾਜਾਨ

ਭੰਡਹੁ ਹੀ ਭੰਡੁ ਊਪਜੈ ਭੰਡੈ ਬਾਝੁ ਨ ਕੋਇ

ਨਾਨਕ ਭੰਡੈ ਬਾਹਰਾ ਏਕੋ ਸਚਾ ਸੋਇ

ਜਿਤੁ ਮੁਖਿ ਸਦਾ ਸਾਲਾਹੀਐ ਭਾਗਾ ਰਤੀ ਚਾਰਿ

ਨਾਨਕ ਤੇ ਮੁਖ ਉਜਲੇ ਤਿਤੁ ਸਚੈ ਦਰਬਾਰਿ ॥2॥

MEHLA PAHELA

Bhand jamee-ai bhand nimee-ai bhand mangan vee-aaho.

Bhandho hovai dostee bhandho chalai raaho

Bhandh muaa bhandh bhaalee-ai bhandh hovai bandhaan

So keo manndaa aakhee-ai jit jameh raajaan

Bhandho hee bhandh oopajai bhandhai baajh na ko-eh

Naanak bhandhai baaharaa ayko sachaa so-eh

Jit mukh sadaa saalaahe-ai bhaagaa ratee chaar.

Naanak tay mukh oojalay tit sachai darbaa-eh (2)

FIRST CHANNEL OF LIGHT, GURU NANAK

From woman, man is born; within woman, man is conceived;
to woman he is engaged and married.
Woman becomes his friend; through woman, the future generations come.
When his woman dies, he seeks another woman; to woman he is bound.
So why call her bad? From her, kings are born.
From woman, woman is born; without woman, there would be no one at all.
O Nanak, only the True Lord is without a woman.
That mouth which praises the Lord continually is blessed and beautiful.
O Nanak, those faces shall be radiant in the Court of the True Lord. ॥ 2 ॥

SOUND MIND & BODY

USING THE SOUND CURRENT
TO CREATE CLARITY & CALIBER

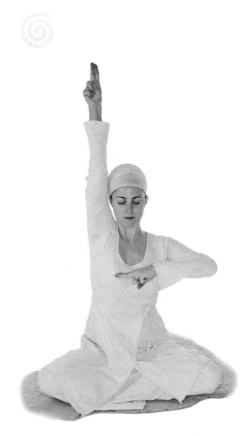

BY CHANTING AND EVOKING the meditative experience of sound through mantra and *shabd*, we each have the capacity to cultivate this strong, solid, and exalted state within ourselves and affect the kind of lasting change in our lives that we so long for.

WHAT DOES EVERY WOMAN WANT IN THIS COMING AGE? To thrive as a woman of grace and divinity, vibrating in highest consciousness! At some point, each of us has experienced a personal sense of alignment with Infinity, reveling in our own inner purity and projecting that purity and light around us. This state comes and goes. But by chanting and evoking the meditative experience of sound through mantra and *shabd*, we each have the capacity to cultivate this strong, solid, and exalted state within ourselves and affect the kind of lasting change in our lives that we so long for.

Among the thousands of rich and profound messages within the Siri Guru Granth Sahib, the living Sikh scriptures and the source of many of the mantras that we use in Kundalini Yoga as taught by Yogi Bhajan®, there is surprisingly only one single command. That command—*Jap*—is found at the very beginning, in the Mul Mantra. *Jap* or *Japa* literally means 'to repeat'. It is the continuous, meditative repetition of a mantra. By repeating mantra in the proper cadence and *naad*—the creative essence—of the mantra, we train the mind in a rich and deep way to vibrate at that frequency, the frequency of the mantra. Bit by bit, our inner reality vibrates with the Infinite reality.

As we continue to chant—to practice *japa*—we create a series of effects in the body and being. Through the action of *japa*, we create *tapa*—divine or psychic heat. This heat then burns the karma—the imprint, or seeds, of past actions (which are also vibrations) that we carry within us. The influence of our karmas can lock us into undesirable habits or shape our current actions and behaviors in unwelcome ways. As the karmas are burnt off and fall away, we find greater freedom and strength to act from a place of consciousness and discipline, rather than impulse and reaction. The end result is dharma—a fulfilled life and a promising future. Yogi Bhajan referred to this progressive effect of *japa* as a simple law—a natural law of the Universe.

Suggestions for Practice

This particular selection of meditations and kriyas uses simple mantras, more complex *shabds* and *banis*, and various postures, breath techniques, mudras and movements to evoke change and create lasting effects. While the approach of each may vary, the end result is rich transformation and a more fulfilled life—all initiated from the simple act of *japa*.

Practicing the simple and powerful **Ganpati Kriya** removes obstacles and makes the impossible possible. With this kriya, you let go of the attachments of the mind and the impact of past actions so that you can live a more creative, dynamic and fulfilled life.

Meditation for an Invincible Spirit instills courage and allows you to overcome the three tendencies of the mind when faced with great change—to be alone & withdrawn, to deny or fantasize about the future that's coming, or to live with greed or scarcity instead of prosperity. This meditation counters these three tendencies and instills the mind with courage and caliber.

Removing the Fear of the Future clears the fears of the future which have been created by your subconscious memories of the past. It allows you to connect to the flow of life through your Heart Center.

Healing the Wounds of Love can be practiced alone or in a group in a uniquely beautiful geometric configuration. Through this practice, you can change your relationships, drop the pain, and strengthen your relationships with clarity, sensitivity and authenticity.

High Tech Yoga allows us to shift gears and respond at a higher frequency to varied circumstances. This practice takes the energy through all of the chakras, allowing us to establish a stronger sense of self.

The practice of **Bowing Jaap Sahib** raises the soul, the self, and the being infusing you with spirit, grit and strength. Use this gift when your grace, your power, and your position are threatened.

DEV SUROOP KAUR KHALSA
ESPAÑOLA, NEW MEXICO

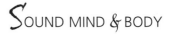

GANPATI KRIYA

JANUARY 1988

POSTURE: Sit in Easy Pose with a straight spine, and a light Neck Lock.

MUDRA: Hands in Gyan Mudra, wrists on the knees, with the arms and elbows straight.

EYE FOCUS: The eyes are 1/10th open. Concentrate at the Third Eye Point.

MANTRA:

> *SAA TAA NAA MAA*
> *RAA MAA DAA SAA*
> *SAA SAY SO HUNG*

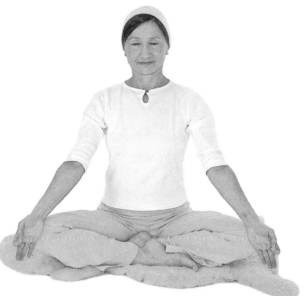

PART ONE

Chant the mantra on a single breath, as you press the fingertips sequentially with each syllable. Use a monotone voice in a Tibetan-like form or use the same melody you would use for Kirtan Kriya.

TIME: Continue for **11-62 minutes**.

PART ONE

Read from Left to Right, chanting the mantra; always begin with the Jupiter finger and end with the little finger.

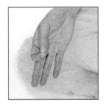 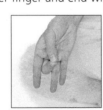 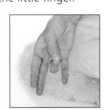 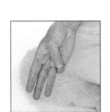

SAA	TAA	NAA	MAA
RAA	MAA	DAA	SAA
SAA	SAY	SO	HUNG

PART TWO

Inhale deeply and suspend the breath. Move the body in a slow twist and stretch motion. Move each muscle of the body. Move the head, torso, arms, back, belly and hands. Then exhale powerfully. Repeat this **3-5 times**.

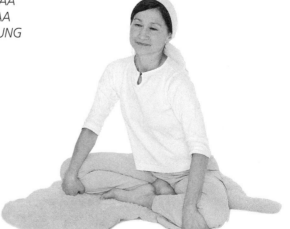

PART TWO

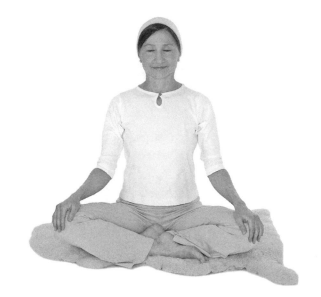

PART THREE

Immediately sit straight. Look at the Lotus Point, the tip of the nose. Become totally calm, absolutely still.
Meditate for **2-3 minutes**.

TO END: Inhale and suspend the breath for 30 seconds as you physically move and rotate the body as if it is going through spasms. Every muscle must be stretched, squeezed and turned around, from the muscles of the face, head and neck, down to the toes. Exhale. Repeat this 3 more times. Then inhale, sit calmly and concentrate on the tip of the nose for 20 seconds. Exhale, and relax.

About This Meditation

This beautiful and powerful meditation has a history in its name. The ancient symbol for this was the Hindu God of Knowledge and Happiness, Ganesha. The other name for Ganesha is *Ganpati*. Ganesha was depicted as a rotund man with the head of an elephant. This huge body balances and rides on a rat, conveying the message that even the impossible can be done with this meditation. The rat represents the quality of penetration. A rat can reach into almost any place. So Ganesha can know anything and can get past any blocks. Wisdom and wise choices grant you happiness in your life.

The impact of this meditation is to clear the blocks from your own karma. Each of us has three regions of life to conquer: First is past which is recorded in our *samskaras* and brings us the challenges and blessings of fate—balanced by these sounds. Second is the present which must be mastered by Karma Yoga—the practice of action with integrity in the moment. Third is the future, recorded in the ether and, which at its best and most fulfilled, is called dharma. This kriya allows you to let go of the attachments of the mind and the impact of past actions so you can create and live a fulfilled life and a perfect future.

MEDITATION TO **REMOVE FEAR OF THE FUTURE**

OCTOBER 26, 1988

POSTURE: Sit comfortably in Easy Pose.

MUDRA: Begin by resting the back of the left hand in the palm of the right hand. Grab the left hand with the right, so that the right thumb nestles in the left palm. Cross the left thumb over the right. The fingers of the right hand curve around the outside of the left hand and hold it gently. Holding your hands in this way will give you a peaceful, secure feeling.

Place this mudra at the Heart Center, resting against the chest.

MANTRA: Meditate to your favorite version of the *shabd*: *Dhan Dhan Ram Das Gur.*

TIME: Start with **11 minutes** and gradually work up to **31 minutes** of practice.

TO END: Inhale deeply and relax.

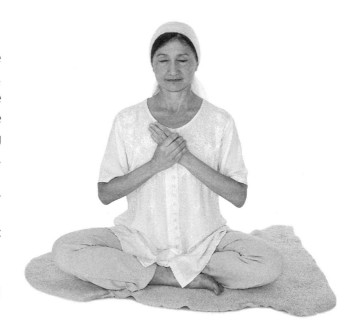

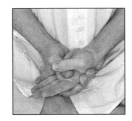

About This Meditation

This meditation clears the fear of the future which has been created by your subconscious memories of the past. It connects you to the flow of life through your Heart Center.

"The beauty in you is your spirit. The strength in you is your endurance. The intelligence in you is your vastness." — Yogi Bhajan

"The crossed thumbs help neutralize your mind's frantic calculations to avoid fear and pain. It is the calculations themselves that produce anxiety and get you out of touch with the resources of your intuition and heart." — Gurucharan Singh Khalsa, Director of Training

HIGH TECH YOGA

JULY 7, 1986

POSTURE: Sit in Easy Pose with a straight spine, and a light Neck Lock.

EYE FOCUS: Eyes are closed.

MANTRA & MUDRA: Chant along with the *Rakhe Rakhanhar* mantra and move in the following sequence of mudras. This is a series of 8 mudras relating to the eight chakras, corresponding to the lines of the mantra. Change at each line of the mantra.

TIME: 127 minutes.

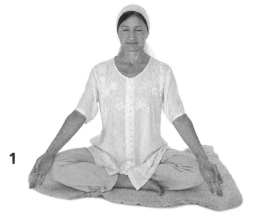

1

Rakhay rakhanhaar aap ubaarian
Gyan Mudra (thumb to index finger):
wrists rest on knees, palms facing outward.

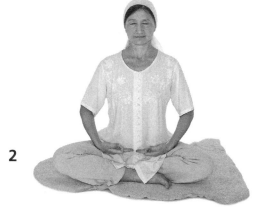

2

Gur kee pairee paa-eh kaaj savaarian
Gyan Mudra: with hands in the lap, palms up.

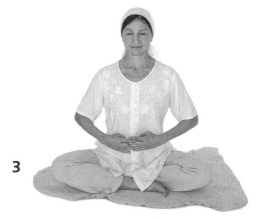

3

Hoaa aap dayaal manho na visaarian
Shuni Mudra (thumb to middle finger):
with fingers pressed at the navel area.

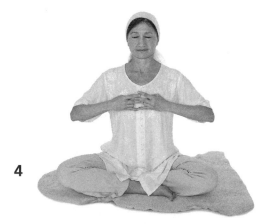

4

Saadh janaa kai sung bhavjal taarian
Surya Mudra (thumb to ring finger):
with fingers pressed at the Heart Center.

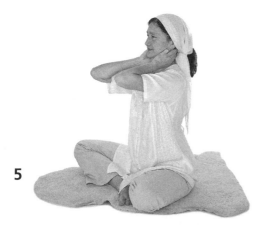

5

Saakat nindak dusht khin maa-eh bidaarian
Buddhi Mudra (thumb to little finger): with fingers pressed below ears facing towards the back of the neck.

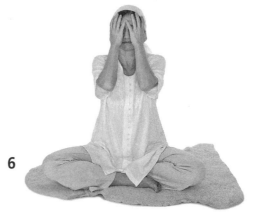

6

Tis saahib kee tayk naanak manai maa-eh
Both hands over the face, fingertips along hairline.

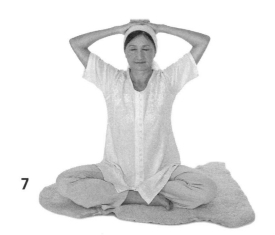

7

Jis simrat sukh ho-eh saglay dookh jaa-eh
Interlock fingers on top of the head.

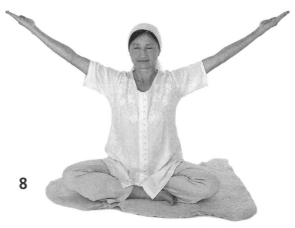

8

Jis simrat sukh ho-eh saglay dookh jaa-eh
Extend arms out straight at 45 degrees with palms up.

About This Meditation

In the face of any great change, we confront three destructive impulses: to be alone and withdrawn, to deny or fantasize about the future that's coming, and to live with greed or scarcity instead of prosperity. This mantra counters these three tendencies and instills the mind with courage and caliber. Focus on the movement of the tongue and the sensation of the sound as it creates a time and space.

Note the subtle difference in the meaning of the words "*Siri*" and "*Maha*." "Great (*Siri*)" still has a touch of finiteness; "Infinite (*Maha*)" has no finiteness or form.

MEDITATION FOR AN INVINCIBLE SPIRIT

FEBRUARY 2, 1992

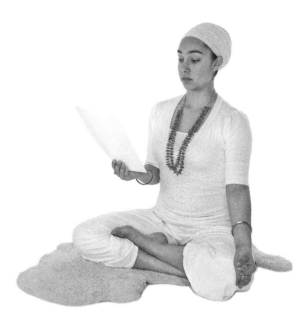

POSTURE: Sit in Easy Pose with a straight spine, and Neck Lock.

MUDRA: Left hand is in Gyan Mudra resting on the knee with the arm straight. Raise the right hand to about 12 inches in front of the chest, holding the mantra sheet and concentrating on the written words as you chant. If you don't have a mantra sheet, angle your hand as if you were reading a sheet of paper, with the palm open and the wrist straight.*

EYE FOCUS: Apply Neck Lock and look down the nose to see the mantra sheet or the palm. When he gave this meditation, Yogi Bhajan asked us to focus the eyes, to pay attention and not drift. If you do not have the page to read from, use the palm but continue to focus.

MANTRA: The mantra is The Mantra for the Aquarian Age.

(a) Chant with Nirinjan Kaur's *Aquarian March*. Become a symphony. **7 minutes** (27 minutes for a 31-minute practice.)

(b) Continue chanting, close the eyes and place the hands on the Heart Center, left palm on the heart, right palm resting on the left hand. Press the hands firmly into the chest. Press hard for **2 minutes**.

(c) Keep your hands on the heart and begin to whisper the mantra. Whisper powerfully. **1 minute**.

(d) Chant without the music for **30 seconds**. Inhale, exhale and relax.

SAT SIREE SIREE AKAAL
Truth, Projective Prosperity and Greatness, Great Undying One Who Knows No Death

SIREE AKAAL MAHAA AKAAL
Great Undying One Who Knows No Death, Infinite Who Is Deathless

MAHAA AKAAL SAT NAAM
Infinite Who Is Deathless, Truth as Identity; or Identity of All That Is

AKAAL MOORAT WHAA-HAY GUROO
Embodied Form or Image of the Infinite, The Ecstatic Totality of God and Existence

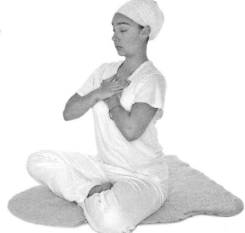

TIME: 11–31 minutes

About This Meditation

In the face of any great change, we confront three destructive impulses: to be alone and withdrawn, to deny or fantasize about the future that's coming, and to live with greed or scarcity instead of prosperity. This mantra counters these three tendencies and instills the mind with courage and caliber. Focus on the movement of the tongue and the sensation of the sound as it creates a time and space.

Note the subtle difference in the meaning of the words "*Siri*" and "*Maha*." "Great (*Siri*)" still has a touch of finiteness; "Infinite (*Maha*)" has no finiteness or form.

* Ideally, you would print the mantra on a sheet of paper and read the mantra as you chant. This is available from KRI for you to download.

HEALING THE WOUNDS OF LOVE

MERA MAN LOCHAI GUR DARSHAN TAA-EE

JULY 7, 1987

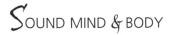
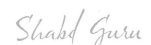

POSTURE: Sit in Easy Pose with a straight spine, and a light Neck Lock.

MANTRA: The first four stanzas of *Shabd Hazaray*, which are the letters wri
by Guru Arjan Dev to Guru Ram Das.

There are four verses that make up this section of *Shabd Hazaray*.
To that sound current we interweave the mantra:

AAD SACH, JUGAAD SACH,
HAIBHAY SACH, NANAK HOSEE BHAI SACH

True in the beginning, True throughout the Ages
True at this moment, Nanak says this Truth shall ever be.

The sequenc of chanting will be:
   Aad Sach Mantra (one time)
   First Letter
   Aad Sach Mantra (one time)
   Second Letter
   Aad Sach Mantra (one time)
   Third Letter
   Aad Sach Mantra (one time)
   Fourth Letter
   Aad Sach Mantra (four times)

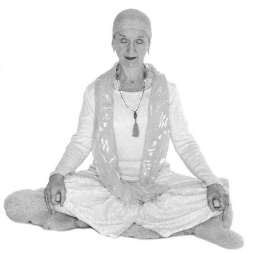

GURU ARJAN DEV, SIRI GURU GRANTH SAHIB, PAGE 96

My mind longs for a sight of my Guru.
It cries out like the thirsty chatrik bird waiting for the rain.
But the rain does not come.
Peace does not come without the sight of my beloved Guru.
I am a sacrifice, my soul is a sacrifice,
Unto the sight of my Beloved Guru. (1)

Your face is so beautiful; hearing your Word brings me deep peace.
It has been so long since this chatrik has seen any water.
O, my dearest friend, O my beloved Guru.
Blessed is the ground beneath your feet.
I am a sacrifice, I am ever a sacrifice
Unto my dearest friend and intimate, my beloved Guru. (2)

Every moment I am away from you a Dark Age dawns for me.
When will I see you, O my beloved Master?
I cannot get through the night without the sight of your Court.
Sleep does not come.
I am a sacrifice, my soul is a sacrifice
Unto the Court of my True Guru. (3)

I am blessed, for I am with my Saintly Guru.
I have found the Eternal God within my own heart/home.
I will serve you every moment of my life, and never be separate from
you again. I am a sacrifice, my soul is a sacrifice unto you.
O my Master, Slave Nanak lives to serve you. (4)

About This Meditation

If you want to change your relationships, drop the pain, empower them with clarity, sensitivity and authenticity, do this meditation **11 times once a day for 11 days**. Of course you can do it each day for as long as you feel necessary or as long as you are enthralled with the beauty and space it creates.

These verses create sound as mantras written in the form of letters between Guru Arjan, the fifth Guru, and Guru Ram Das, his father, the fourth Guru. There was perfect longing, love and fulfillment in the sentiments, feelings, projection and elevation of these letters. Repeating these mantras takes you out of the normal internal chatter and emotional games of the mind we usually live with. It purifies, aligns and strengthens the heart and soul.

THE FOUR LETTERS OF GURU ARJAN TO GURU RAM DAS
FROM SHABD HAZARAY
Guru Arjan Dev, Siri Guru Granth Sahib, page 96

Aad sach, jugaad such, haibhai sach,
nanak hosee bhai sach

F I R S T
Mayraa man lochai gur darshan taa-ee
Bilap karay chaatrik kee ni-aa-ee
Trikhaa na utarai shaant na aavai
Bin Darshan Sant pi-aaray jee-o
Hao gholee jee-o ghol ghumaa-ee
Gur darshan sant pi-aaray jee-o (1)

Aad sach, jugaad sach, haibhai sach,
nanak hosee bhai sach

S E C O N D
Tayraa mukh suhaavaa jee-o sahaj dhun baanee
Chir ho-aa daykhay saaring paanee
Dhan so days jahaa too(n) vasi-aa
Mayray sajan meet muraaray jee-o
Hao gholee hao ghol ghumaa-ee
Gur sajan meet muraaray jee-o (2)

Aad sach, jugaad sach, haibhai sach,
nanak hosee bhai sach

T H I R D
Ik gharee na milatay taa kalijug hotaa
Hun kad milee-ai pri-a tudh bhagavantaa
Mo-eh rain na vihaavai need na aavai
Bin daykhay gur darbaaray jee-o
Hao gholee jee-o ghol ghumaa-ee
Tis sachay gur darbaaray jee-o (3)

Aad sach, jugaad sach, haibhai sach,
nanak hosee bhai sach

F O U R T H
Bhaag ho-aa gur sant milaa-i-aa
Prabh abinaasee ghar meh paa-i-aa
Sayv karee pal chasaa na vichhuraa
Jan Naanak daas tumaaray jee-o
Hao gholee jee-o ghol ghumaa-ee
Jan Naanak daas tumaaray jee-o (4)

Aad sach, jugaad sach, haibhai sach, nanak hosee bhai sach
Aad sach, jugaad sach, haibhai sach, nanak hosee bhai sach
Aad sach, jugaad sach, haibhai sach, nanak hosee bhai sach
Aad sach, jugaad sach, haibhai sach, nanak hosee bhai sach

ਮੇਰਾ ਮਨ ਲੋਚੈ ਗੁਰ ਦਰਸਨ ਤਾਈ
ਬਲਪ ਕਰੇ ਚਾਤ੍ਰਿਕ ਕੀ ਨਿਆਈ
ਤ੍ਰਿਖਾ ਨ ਉਤਰੈ ਸਾਂਤਿ ਨ ਆਵੈ
ਬਿਨ ਦਰਸਨ ਸੰਤ ਪਿਆਰੇ ਜੀਉ ॥ 1 ॥
ਹਉ ਘੋਲੀ ਜੀਉ ਘੋਲਿ ਘੁਮਾਈ
ਗੁਰ ਦਰਸਨ ਸੰਤ ਪਿਆਰੇ ਜੀਉ ॥ 1 ॥

ਤੇਰਾ ਮੁਖੁ ਸੁਹਾਵਾ ਜੀਉ ਸਹਜ ਧੁਨਿ ਬਾਣੀ
ਚਿਰੁ ਹੋਆ ਦੇਖੇ ਸਾਰਿੰਗਪਾਣੀ
ਧੰਨੁ ਸੁ ਦੇਸੁ ਜਹਾ ਤੂੰ ਵਸਿਆ
ਮੇਰੇ ਸਜਣ ਮੀਤ ਮੁਰਾਰੇ ਜੀਉ ॥ 2 ॥
ਹਉ ਘੋਲੀ ਹਉ ਘੋਲਿ ਘੁਮਾਈ
ਗੁਰ ਸਜਣ ਮੀਤ ਮੁਰਾਰੇ ਜੀਉ ॥ 1 ॥

ਇਕ ਘੜੀ ਨ ਮਿਲਤੇ ਤਾ ਕਲਿਜੁਗੁ ਹੋਤਾ
ਹੁਨਿ ਕਦਿ ਮਿਲੀਐ ਪ੍ਰਿਅ ਤੁਧੁ ਭਗਵੰਤਾ
ਮੋਹਿ ਰੈਨਿ ਨ ਵਿਹਾਵੈ ਨੀਦ ਨ ਆਵੈ
ਬਿਨੁ ਦੇਖੇ ਗੁਰ ਦਰਬਾਰੇ ਜੀਉ ॥ 3 ॥

ਹਉ ਘੋਲੀ ਜੀਉ ਘੋਲਿ ਘੁਮਾਈ
ਤਿਸੁ ਸਚੇ ਗੁਰ ਦਰਬਾਰੇ ਜੀਉ ॥ 1 ॥
ਭਾਗੁ ਹੋਆ ਗੁਰਿ ਸੰਤੁ ਮਿਲਾਇਆ
ਪ੍ਰਭੁ ਅਬਿਨਾਸੀ ਘਰ ਮਹਿ ਪਾਇਆ
ਸੇਵ ਕਰੀ ਪਲੁ ਚਸਾ ਨ ਵਿਛੁੜਾ
ਜਨ ਨਾਨਕ ਦਾਸ ਤੁਮਾਰੇ ਜੀਉ ॥ 4 ॥
ਹਉ ਘੋਲੀ ਜੀਉ ਘੋਲਿ ਘੁਮਾਈ
ਜਨ ਨਾਨਕ ਦਾਸ ਤੁਮਾਰੇ ਜੀਉ ॥ 1 ॥ 8 ॥

BOWING JAAP SAHIB
GURBANI OF GURU GOBIND SINGH

POSTURE: Sit on the heels in Rock Pose, with hands on thighs.

MANTRA: Recitation of Guru Gobind Singh's *Jaap Sahib*.

MOVEMENT: Begin bowing the forehead to the floor to the *Namastang* rhythm:

With the recitation:
Bowing 4 counts, resting 1 with the music.
(Consider one cycle of touching the forehead to the floor and rising as 1 count.)

Without the recitation:
The movement is done to 10 beats as follows:
Down on 1, Up on 2, Down on 3, Up on 4, Down on 5, Up on 6, Down on 7, Up on 8. Stay up for beats 9 and 10.

ALTERNATIVE MUDRA: This can also be done with the arms and hands in **Yoga Mudra**: hands interlaced at the base of the spine, palms facing up. Arms would stretch up as high as possible when the forehead touches the ground.

TIME: Continue for the entire recitation of the *Jaap Sahib*.

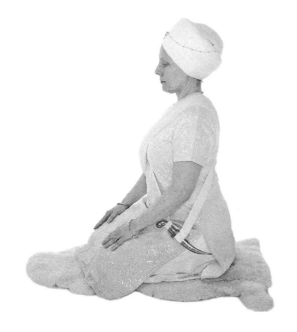

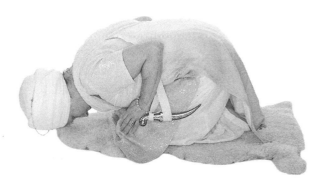

About Bowing Jaap Sahib

"*Jaap Sahib* is Guru Gobind Singh's *bani*, it comes from the third center of balanced naad. So that we would not become beggars at the doors of others and be insulted, Guru Gobind Singh became one with God and recited *Jaap Sahib*. You have to understand: the Sikhs of Guru Gobind Singh were in a position to run at the speed of a horse. What was the miracle that gave them such power? *Jaap Sahib*. *Jaap Sahib* gives you the strength of mind behind every muscle of you. And if we have to face challenge or change, take the Name of God everywhere, with every breath. This is how we can do it. That is the way to be spiritual. Everything you do should be right from your spirit, and your spirit should be in it. That's the way you can succeed. Nothing else will work it out.

That's why he recited *Jaap Sahib*. This *bani* is a gift to you to use when your grace, your power, and your position are threatened. Whoever will recite this *bani* shall never fall flat on his face. That's why an ordinary bunch of bones could fight with thousands and thousands of armed, trained soldiers and defend themselves beautifully; because they had the spirit with them.

Jaap Sahib is not just to praise God. To praise God is the way we have been taught. It's the oldest method, because man wanted to be with God and so he was told to pray and meditate. That is where I differ. I have experienced and I believe that these things are there to make us highly sensitive, absolutely creative and extremely intuitive. It doesn't matter how rich you are, how healthy you are or how good you are. It doesn't matter if you have all the faculties of life which you want to have. If you are not intuitive, you are dumb. That's how pain comes, I am trying to take you past that. For that you need new blood. That's why we are doing these exercises, so that the glands can work.

Jaap Sahib is the salutation to God in which Guru Gobind Singh recites every facet of God. As many facets as have been explained there, that many facets you have to cover in your life. That's what *Jaap Sahib* is. But to do that, you require about 250 years to learn, practice, experience and project each facet. I don't think we have that time. So basically, the idea of the mantra is to give you the key to open that hemisphere where you want to be. That's what *Jaap Sahib* does. When you do it in this bowing form, it will keep you healthy, happy and holier than you can imagine. You can enjoy life.

If you want to live with your hurts, and continue to cause yourself the hurts, that is a different science and a different theory. As far as I am concerned, no woman is meant to be hurt. I think that basically, we should not tolerate that. It is my feeling that if we really work hard on ourselves and flow with our own energy. we can penetrate through life successfully. Expecting somebody else to help you or to make you happy or feel good is asking for trouble. Rather, you should make yourself so happy that by looking at you, people should become happy. You do not understand your basics. Whether you are married or not, have children or not, you have to keep the entire dimension, the entire domain happy—that's a woman's work. For a woman to reach God is as easy as for me to go from here to my ranch.

So, when victory came, Guru Gobind Singh praised the Lord in naad. That is what is beautiful about *Jaap Sahib*: it raises the soul and the Self, the being. And that is what we are talking about. I'm just trying to give you the experience as I learned Gurbani, and as I learned Kundalini Yoga.

Mimick this *Jaap Sahib*. You are not mimicking the words, you are recreating the creative essence of the word, the naad. This is a powerful way that you can learn about sensitivity. If you can practice this meditatively, then whatever people say, you will always compute what people mean. It will give you a totally different dimension. It will take away unawareness, foolishness and nonsense. What a person is saying and what he actually means are two different dimensions. And that is what I want you to experience.

—Yogi Bhajan

Part Two

WOMAN IS INVINCIBLE

Healer ○ *Leader* ○ *Nurturer*

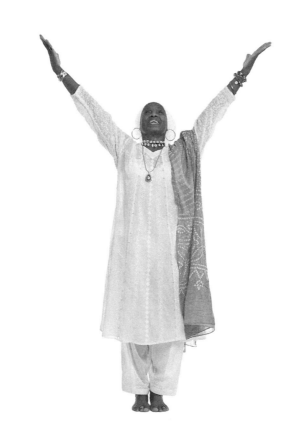

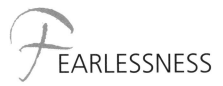

FEARLESSNESS

EMPOWER YOUR LIFE

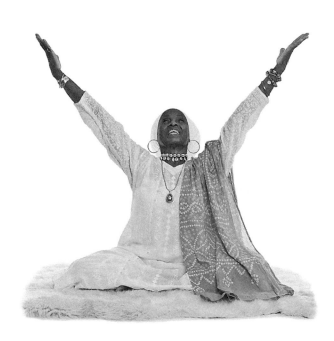

THE FIRST STEP TOWARD FEARLESSNESS is to let go of the past by locating your Self in the brilliant clarity of stillness we call our soul or Higher Self.

ESSENTIAL KRIYAS FOR WOMEN IN THE AQUARIAN AGE

IN TODAY'S CULTURE, EMPOWERMENT IS SPOKEN of so often, it's become somewhat of a cliché. In truth, it can be extremely elusive for a woman, if she does not create it from within. Yet, a woman who's empowered to be herself, to be respected, to be honored—can still change the world. Fearlessness is a quality of the divine—*nirbho*. What does fearlessness mean in the life of a woman, a mother, a sister, a wife? Each of these roles is rife with insecurity and attachment. The very physiology of the women seems to make her vulnerable; woman is wired to be insecure. And her roles demand a level of attachment that is hard to break. Actually, she's wired to be sensitive. She's wired to protect and secure her surroundings. So what does fearlessness look like? For a woman to be truly fearless, she has to let go of attachment and ego, and she has to learn to trust. This is the great paradox and the great struggle.

Most women at some point in their life have been abused—verbally, sexually, physically, even energetically. For a woman to walk through life constantly accosted or in fear of it, the notion of fearlessness seems beside the point. But the first step toward fearlessness is to let go of the past by locating your Self in the brilliant clarity of stillness we call our soul or Higher Self. Then, expand that Self to connect and rely on the Infinite God. From this platform, we learn to embrace the world anew with love and fearless wisdom; we learn to trust in God within and without. Those who've been abused in the past, especially by people who were supposed to protect them, find this one of the most challenging aspects of transforming themselves from victim to victor. Blame and shame often leave a very deep imprint. But leaving the past behind and trusting in the flow of life is the beginning of fearlessness.

As we clear the past, and strengthen and relax into our essence through Kundalini Yoga as taught by Yogi Bhajan®, our intuition becomes more accurate and we begin to perceive our inner guidance as something we can actually trust. The contraction and restriction of fear is gradually reversed, and we begin to truly explore and apply our talent and potential in all that we do. In the process of letting go of fear, you may find as I did, that layers of depression or anger may release first, keep pressing on. Your deepest fears will be cleared as well.

THE KRIYAS AND MEDITATIONS in this chapter can take you from fear and anxiety to power and integrity. They build vitality, strong nerves, and a powerful Navel Point, which gives you identity and courage. **Outward Bound** is one of my personal favorites; it prepares you to meet the world head on—vibrant and strong. Because our female reproductive system is totally internal, we require vigorous, daily exercise, in order to have enough extroverted energy to really excel and work in today's world. This set is a perfect example of bring that internal energy out.

The **Kriya to Relax and Release Fear** works on the glands and the organs to move stagnant energy in the liver, which can help to release anger, and then stimulates the kidneys, which are associated with fear. It also incorporates **Bowing Jaap Sahib**, which builds stamina and courage. Each of the meditations tonifies your nervous system by using the breath, the *prana*, alleviating depression and lethargy and building vitality and stamina.

The *25th pauri of Japji Sahib* is an amazing gift that I have used for decades to build prosperity, whenever I walk. Its sound current helps to attract to you what you need without asking! It contains the two-line sutra that Yogi Bhajan said was the sutra of his life: "*Kayti-aa Dookh Bhookh Sad Maar, Ayeh Bhi Daat Teyree Daataar.*" Its meaning is "So many are continually beaten down by endless pain and hunger. Even these are Your gifts to us, Great Giver." (Translation by Ek Ong Kaar Kaur).

If you meditate on the sound current of Infinity with each breath, instead of allowing the mind to continually expound on its worries and manipulations, the universe will assist you through every test, and grant you an attitude of gratitude, which is the ultimate manifestation of grace on this Earth.

DEVA KAUR KHALSA
CORAL SPRINGS, FLORIDA
& SAT PURKH KAUR KHALSA
ESPAÑOLA, NEW MEXICO

KRIYA TO **RELAX & RELEASE FEAR**
ORIGINALLY FROM KUNDALINI YOGA FOR YOUTH AND JOY

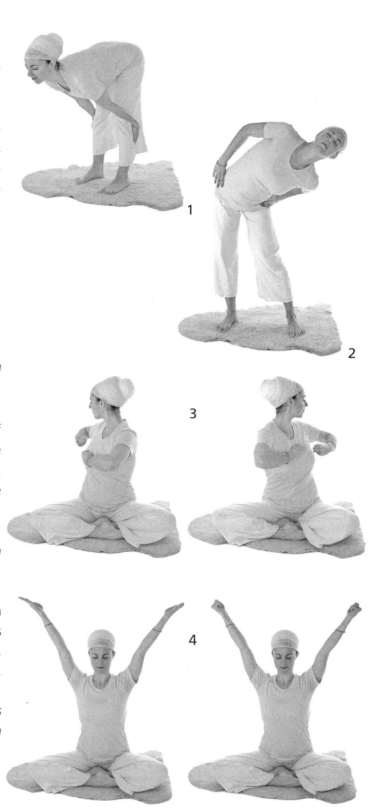

1. Stand Up. Bend forward from the waist, keeping the back parallel to the ground. Grab the calves or behind the knees. Begin to flex the spine as in Cat/Cow Posture. Inhale and flex the spine downwards as if someone were sitting on your back. When the spine is pressed downwards the neck is arched up. Exhale and flex the spine in the opposite direction, bringing the chin to the chest. Use the hands and feet as a firm base of support for the spine. The legs remain straight. Continue with a steady rhythm, coordinating the movement with the breath. **7 minutes**. *This exercise works on the kidneys and liver.*

2. Remain standing and place the hands on the hips. Rapidly rotate the torso in large circles from the waist. Continue this twisting motion powerfully for **9 minutes**. *This exercise rejuvenates the spleen and liver. You may feel nauseous as the liver releases toxins.*

3. Sit in Easy Pose. Make fists and place them in front of you as if grasping a steering wheel. Begin twisting the body powerfully from side to side. Twist to your maximim. Keep the elbows up and let the neck move also. Inhale left, exhale right, with a powerful breath.
Continue for **4 minutes**.
This exercise works on the kidneys. The neck must move in order to release the blood supply to the brain.

4. Remain sitting in Easy Pose. Extend the arms up at a 60° angle, palms facing up, fingers straight and thumbs extended out. Begin to open and close the hands rapidly, bringing the tips of the fingers to the base of the palms. Continue for **7 minutes**.
This exercise breaks up deposits in the fingers and prevents arthritis. If you already have arthritis, it may work on improving it.

5. Sit in Easy Pose. Extend the arms out to the sides parallel to the ground. Make fists of the hands with the thumbs tucked inside the hands touching the fleshy mound below the little finger. Inhale through the mouth and flex the elbows, bringing the fists to the shoulders. As you exhale through the mouth, straighten the arms out to the sides. Move rapidly and breathe powerfully. Stiffen the mouth into an "O" as you inhale and exhale. Continue rhythmically, coordinating the movement with the breath for **6 minutes**.

This exercise removes tension from the neck and purifies the blood. In this exercise your fears will leave you when you powerfully project out on the exhale.

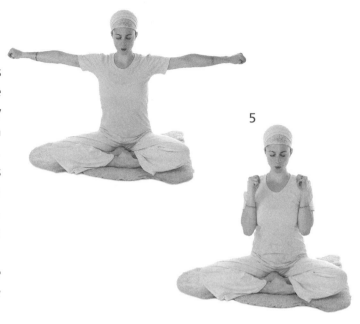

6. Still in Easy Pose, begin rotating the fists in small circles at the level of the Heart Center—left fist counter clockwise; right fist clockwise. Keep the elbows straight and fists tight. Move the shoulder blades and the muscles underneath the shoulder area. Continue powerfully for **2 minutes**.

This exercise adjusts the muscles under the breasts. If this area is tight, it makes you very uptight.

7. Crouch in **Crow Pose**, soles of the feet flat on the floor, with the knees wide, and drawn up towards the chest. Keep the spine straight. Make fists of the hands with the thumbs out, and place them near your neck just above the shoulders. Fists stay in this position as you inhale and stand up. Exhale and lower yourself back down to Crow Pose. Continue for **3 minutes**.

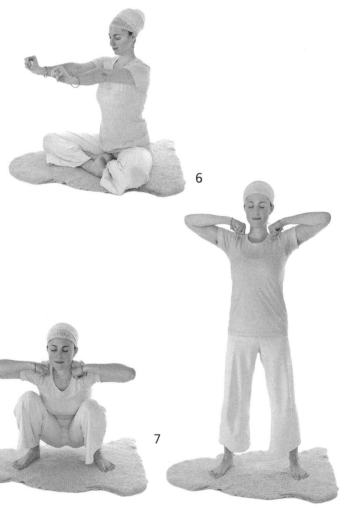

8. **Sitali Pranayam**. Sit in Easy Pose and relax the hands on the knees. Keep the spine straight. Curl the tongue and protrude it slightly past the lips. Inhale deeply and smoothly through the tongue and mouth. Exhale through the nose. Make the breath long and heavy. After **4-5 minutes**, play the *Dukh Bhanjan* recording if available*, and meditate on the healing vibrations of the Golden Temple[1] and the *shabd* (sound current of the words). Continue breathing rhythmically, coordinating the breath to the music. Continue for **2 minutes**.

Sitali Pranayam is effective against anger, bad moods and temperament. If your mouth becomes bitter, it means you have bad breath, but it is being cleaned out as you do this pranayam. This shabd, Dukh Bhanjan was sung in praise of that place where many were healed by a sip and dip in the nectar tank at the Golden Temple.

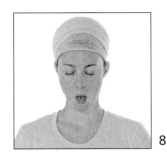

8

9. Continue listening to the recording. Sit in Easy Pose and raise the arms, curving them upwards. Close your eyes and rhythmically move your body to the music. Move as your body feels. Stop thinking and move with the beat. If you can bring your body into exact rhythm with the music, you can go into a state of ecstacy. Continue for **10 minutes**.

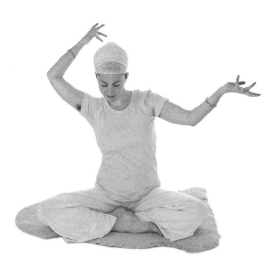

9

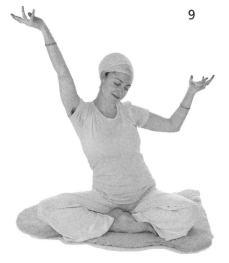

10. **Bowing Jaap Sahib**. Sit on the heels in Rock Pose, with hands on thighs. Listen to a recording of *Jaap Sahib* and begin bowing the forehead to the floor to the *Namastang* rhythm:

Bowing 4 counts. Resting 1 with the music.

(Touching the forehead to the ground and rising up is 1 count.)

Without the recording the movement is done to 10 beats as follows: Bow down and come up 4 times (to the count of 8) and rest in the upward position, on counts 9 and 10. Continue for **8 minutes**.

This exercise done in Rock Pose has been known to heal any rock formations in the body such as kidney stones and gallstones.

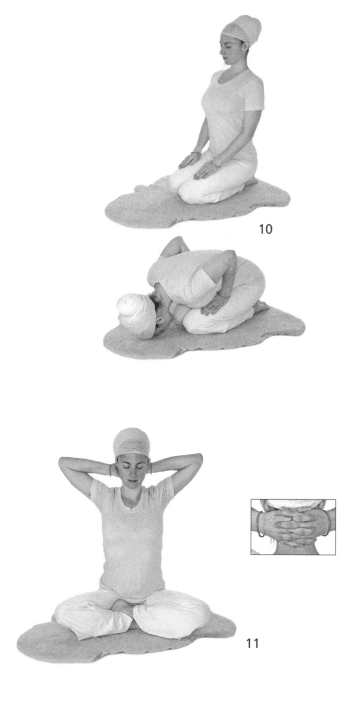

10

11. Sit in a meditative posture. Lock the hands behind the back of the head in Venus Lock, elbows out to the sides and apply pressure, keeping the spine straight. Close your eyes and begin chanting aloud with the *Jaap Sahib* recording. Copy the very essence of it and feel the vibrations going through your hands to the back of the head as you chant. If the recording is not available, breathe long and gently in this position. Continue **8 minutes**. Relax.

Let yourself become calm and together. Feel that you are going to achieve God's Light in you. Totally remove any difference between yourself and God.

11

[1] This refers to the Golden Temple, or Harimandir Sahib, in Amritsar, India. This is a great healing place of the Sikhs, which welcomes all people.

* Other beautiful recordings are available which invoke the experience of the Golden Temple. A few are: Pritpal SIngh's recording *Prayer for the Golden Temple*, Guru Raj Kaur's *Narayan*, or Sat Kartar's *Har Har Amritsar.*

MEDITATION TO **TOTALLY RECHARGE YOU**

OCTOBER 3, 1979

POSTURE: Sit in Easy Pose with a straight spine, and a light Neck Lock.

MUDRA: Extend the arms straight out in front, parallel to the ground. Close the right hand into a fist. Wrap the left fingers around the right fist. The base of the palms touch, thumbs are extended up and touch along the sides.

EYE FOCUS: The eyes are focused on the thumbs.

BREATHE: Inhale for **5 seconds**. Exhale for **5 seconds**. Suspend the breath out for **15 seconds**. Continue.

TIME: Start with **3-5 minutes** and work up to **11 minutes** Build up the time slowly. In time, you can work up to holding the breath out for 1 full minute.

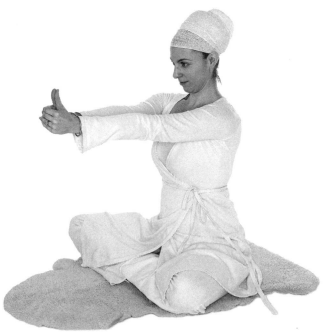

About This Meditation

This meditation totally recharges you. It is an antidote to depression. It builds a new system, gives you the capacity and caliber to deal with life, and gives you a direct relationship with your pranic body.

OUTWARD BOUND KRIYA

MAY 3, 1984

1. **Leg Lift Variation**. Lie flat on the back. Lift one leg to 90 degrees. Keeping it raised, lift the other leg up to 45 degrees. Bring them both down at the same time. Switch legs and repeat. **11 minutes**.
This brings healing to your entire "apana" area: gonads, pelvis and uterus, and is very important for women.

2. **Plow Pose**. Lie flat with hands extended over the head on the ground. Raise the legs up over the head, and bring them back down. **52 times**.

3. **Frog Pose Variation**. Begin in Frog Pose, squatting, with both hands touching the ground in front. As you extend the hips up, bring the left hand to the heart. Then settle back down in Frog Pose, both hands on the ground. Extend up again and bring the right hand to the heart, and then squat back down, both hands back on the ground. Alternate. The heels remain off the ground. Continue in a brisk fashion. **54 times**.

4. **Forward Bends**. Standing up, inhale and reach the arms up to the sky. Exhale, bend over at the waist and touch the ground. Continue **54 times**.

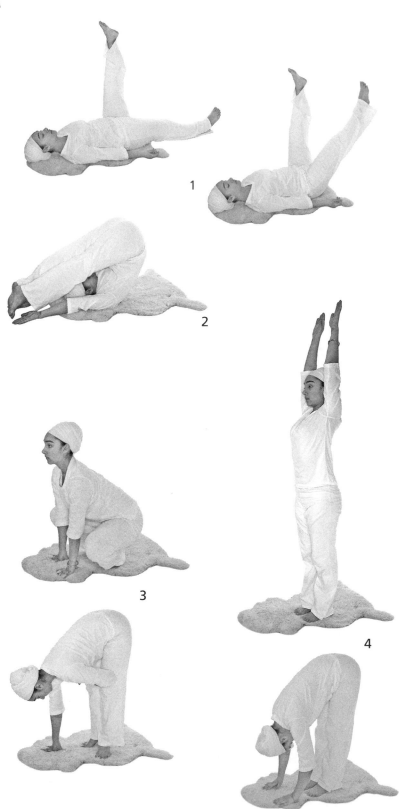

5. **Front Stretch Variation**. Sit with the legs stretched out front. Lengthening the spine, grab the feet, bending forward from the navel, bringing the torso toward the knees. Hold this posture and roll the neck around in a circle. **52 circles**.

6. **Bow Pose**. Lying flat on the stomach, reach back and grab the ankles. Inhale and stretch upwards into Bow Pose, arching the head back. Exhale and relax the thighs and head down to the ground. Breathe powerfully. **74 times**.

7. **Deep Relaxation**. Lie flat on the back and relax the entire body to the sound of Gong (if available.) Yogi Bhajan played the Nobility song as the last part of the relaxation.

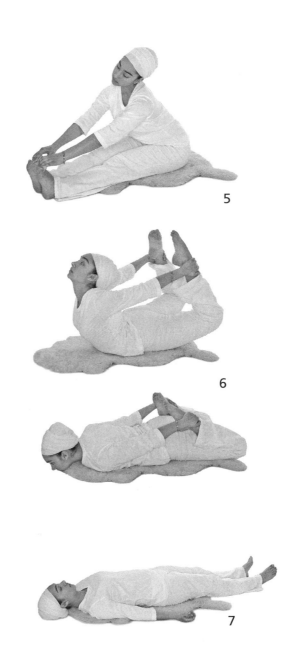

About This Kriya

"A woman needs one to two hours of tough exercise each day in order to be as productive as a man. Every 72 hours the cells change, but in the case of a woman, it needs to be accelerated or stimulated to do so. By nature, a woman in her child-bearing capacity, is very inward. To remain outward, she is required to exercise. You must exercise in a way that stimulates all parts of you. To keep your body young and healthy is your challenge. It cannot be done by makeup. It can only be done by intensive exercise. The principle of life is to meditate in the evening, and to exercise at least one hour every day."   — Yogi Bhajan

MEDITATION FOR **STRONG NERVES**

SEPTEMBER 29, 1975

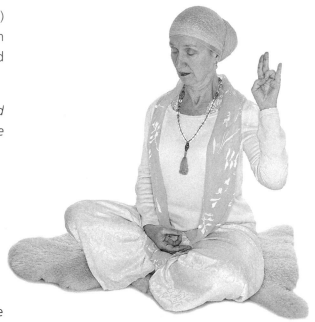

POSTURE: Sit in Easy Pose with a straight spine, and a light Neck Lock.

MUDRA: Left hand is in Ravi Mudra (thumb tip and Sun (ring) finger touch; fingernails don't touch) at the level of the ear, palm facing forward. The right hand is in Buddhi Mudra (thumb tip and Mercury (little) finger touching, resting in the lap, palm up.

(Males reverse the position so that the right hand has thumb and ring finger touching, hand at ear level, and the left hand is in the lap with the thumb and little finger touching.)

EYE FOCUS: The eyes are 1/10 open.

BREATH: Make the breath long and deep.

TIME: Start with **11 minutes** and work up to 31 minutes.

TO END: Inhale deeply, raise the arms up overhead, open the fingers wide, and shake them rapidly for several minutes. Relax.

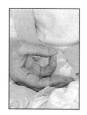 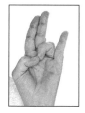

About This Meditation

This is one of five meditations taught by Yogi Bhajan specifically to prepare for "the grey period of the planet and to bring mental balance." Practice this meditation to gain a calm mind and strong nerves. It will help protect you from irrational behavior.

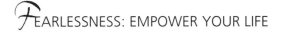

MEDITATION FOR **MENTAL CONTROL**
BRAHM KALAA KRIYA

POSTURE: Sit in Easy Pose with a straight spine, and a light Neck Lock.

EYE FOCUS: Eyes are closed.

MUDRA: Cross the arms in front of the chest. Elbows bent at 90 degrees, arms parallel to the ground. Place the right palm on top of the left upper arm. The top of the left hand rests under the right upper arm. Fingers are together and straight. Balance this posture, and stretch the arms out from the shoulders as much possible.

BREATH: The breath will become very slow.

TIME: Begin with **3 minutes** and gradually increase to **11 minutes**.

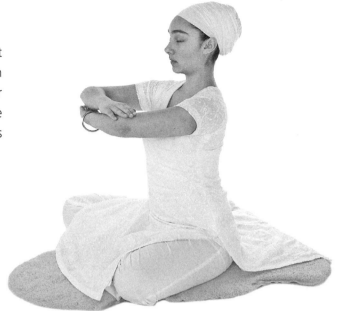

About This Meditation

Kalaa is another name for Kundalini. In this kriya, it's as though you were extending your Self out into the Universe. The practice of Brahm Kalaa can give you control over your own death.

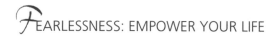

BEING IN THE FLOW
THE 25TH PAURI OF JAPJI SAHIB

Shabd Guru

"When the sun comes out of the clouds, everything is lit. When the mind comes out of duality, prosperity is there. The 25th Pauri of Japji Sahib has the power to take away duality because it covers every aspect of the projected self and its radiance. It works on the Tenth Body, the Radiant Body, which is how prosperity is produced. Those people who have never seen richness, who have nothing, if they read this pauri 11 times a day, they'll become incredibly prosperous."

—Yogi Bhajan, March 20, 1984

"If you recite the 25th Pauri 11 times a day, you can never be poor, even if you are insane. If you are a certified lunatic, you'll still be rich. The vibration of that pauri is par excellent. Why? Because this pauri cuts out your karma, gives you applied consciousness and brings you everything that is in the psyche. If you bless somebody, he'll become the king of the kings. Nanak recited this pauri to cut down karma— and not only karma, but also to cut down samskaras, which carry the vibration of the previous life."

—Yogi Bhajan, September 19, 1989

Normally, we are taught, and most of us still believe, that prosperity is the result of what we do. From a yogic perspective, however, prosperity comes through our radiance and our projected consciousness. As we vibrate, so we attract; as we glow, so we grow.

When the 25th *Pauri* is recited with devotion and focus 11 times a day, it raises our vibratory frequency and develops our radiance so that we attract the best things in life. But how does it work? It works through the science of reversal. In the 25th *Pauri*, Guru Nanak describes the most difficult situations that a soul can go through: people who have wasted their lives through vice; people who take everything and then deny that they have anything; people who suffer countless hungers and beatings. Psychologically, what Guru Nanak describes is very challenging. But then he takes this vision, he takes these souls living their tragic lives, and he gives them back to the Creator. "Even these experiences are Your gifts to us, Great Giver," Guru Nanak says. It's a 180-degree turn.

In the 25th *Pauri*, the mind is asked to acknowledge every experience, no matter how terrible, as a gift from the Creator to the soul. When the mind begins to vibrate with this perspective, then the entire Universe, and everything contained within it, is seen as pure abundance. When we relate to everything as a gift, it grows within us the spirit of gratitude and appreciation. When that attitude of gratitude and appreciation vibrates from the center of our being, then all we need will come to us. The attitude of gratitude, even in the most difficult and terrible experiences, cuts through the karmas and the blocks, and takes the mind out of its duality, allowing us to flow with the abundant nature of the Divine.

Reciting the 25th *Pauri* 11 times a day will work whether you completely understand what the words mean or not. It is a prayer of gratitude, it is a prayer of surrender, it is a prayer of acceptance, it is a prayer of praise. It will awaken in you the experience of your own radiance, your own capacity to magnetize what you need from Infinity through the purity of your own Being.

EK ONG KAAR KAUR KHALSA
ESPAÑOLA, NEW MEXICO

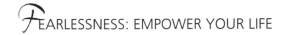

BEING IN THE FLOW
THE 25TH PAURI OF JAPJI SAHIB

ਬਹੁਤਾ ਕਰਮੁ ਲਿਖਿਆ ਨਾ ਜਾਇ ॥ ਵਡਾ ਦਾਤਾ ਤਿਲੁ ਨ ਤਮਾਇ

ਕੇਤੇ ਮੰਗਹਿ ਜੋਧ ਅਪਾਰ ॥ ਕੇਤਿਆ ਗਣਤ ਨਹੀ ਵੀਚਾਰੁ

ਕੇਤੇ ਖਪਿ ਤੁਟਹਿ ਵੇਕਾਰ ॥ ਕੇਤੇ ਲੈ ਲੈ ਮੁਕਰੁ ਪਾਹਿ

ਕੇਤੇ ਮੂਰਖ ਖਾਹੀ ਖਾਹਿ

ਕੇਤਿਆ ਦੂਖ ਭੂਖ ਸਦ ਮਾਰ

ਏਹਿ ਭਿ ਦਾਤਿ ਤੇਰੀ ਦਾਤਾਰ

ਬੰਦਿ ਖਲਾਸੀ ਭਾਣੈ ਹੋਇ ॥ ਹੋਰੁ ਆਖਿ ਨ ਸਕੈ ਕੋਇ

ਜੇ ਕੋ ਖਾਇਕੁ ਆਖਣਿ ਪਾਇ ॥ ਓਹੁ ਜਾਣੈ ਜੇਤੀਆ ਮੁਹਿ ਖਾਇ

ਆਪੇ ਜਾਣੈ ਆਪੇ ਦੇਇ ॥ ਆਖਹਿ ਸਿ ਭਿ ਕੇਈ ਕੇਇ

ਜਿਸ ਨੋ ਬਖਸੇ ਸਿਫਤਿ ਸਾਲਾਹ

ਨਾਨਕ ਪਾਤਿਸਾਹੀ ਪਾਤਿਸਾਹੁ ॥੨੫॥

Bahuta karam likhiaa na jaa-ay. Vadaa dataa til na tamaay.

Kaytay mange jodh apaar. Kaythiaa ganat nahee veechaar.

Kaytay khap tuteh vekar. Kaytay lai lai mukar paa-eh.

Kaytay moorakh khaahee khaa-eh.

Kaytiaa dookh bhookh sad maar.

Ay-eh bhe daat tayree daataar.

Band khaalasee bhanai hoe. Hor aakh na sakai koe.

Jay ko khaa-ik akhaan paae. Oh jaanai jaytee-aa muh khaa-ay.

Aapay jaanay aapay day-eh. Aakheh se bhe kay-ee kay-eh.

Jis no bakhsay siphat saalaah.

Naanak paatisaahee paatisaah.

His Blessings are so abundant that there can be no written account of them.

The Great Giver does not hold back anything.

There are so many great, heroic warriors begging at the Door of the Infinite Lord.

So many contemplate and dwell upon Him, that they cannot be counted.

So many waste away to death engaged in corruption.

So many take and take again, and then deny receiving.

So many foolish consumers keep on consuming.

So many endure distress, deprivation and constant abuse.

Even these are Your Gifts, O Great Giver! Liberation from bondage comes only by Your Will.

No one else has any say in this. If some fool should presume to say that he does,

he shall learn, and feel the effects of his folly. He Himself knows, He Himself gives.

Few, very few are those who acknowledge this.

One who is blessed to sing the Praises of the Lord, O Nanak, is the king of kings. ‖ 25 ‖

ਬਹੁਤਾ ਕਰਮੁ ਲਿਖਿਆ ਨਾ ਜਾਇ ਵਡਾ ਦਾਤਾ ਤਿਲੁ ਨ ਤਮਾਇ

WOMAN AS HER OWN PSYCHOLOGIST I

CLEARING THE SELF

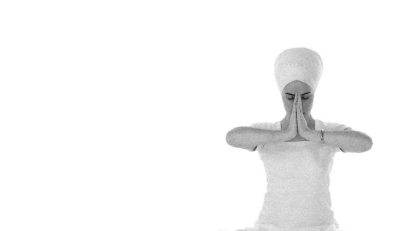

AWAKEN THE INTUITIVE MIND and draw upon your deep intelligence and rewrite your destiny on a cellular level. Through our practice we develop the patience to recognize our past, appreciate it for the gifts it delivered, bless it—and then drop it!

ESSENTIAL KRIYAS FOR WOMEN IN THE AQUARIAN AGE

AS WOMEN WE FACE AN AMAZING CHALLENGE and opportunity, in our lives. Yogi Bhajan said that our biological, physiological, sociological and mental capacity is 16 times greater than a man's, provided we explore it. This is truly an incredible gift and yet with this gift comes an incredible responsibility because every woman has "16 times the power to destroy herself or build herself."

So often we face our challenges beautifully. We meditate, we pray, we align ourselves with the divine and we excel. Then there are those times when we are not tuning in to our Higher Self and someone or something else seems to be in control. Our language feels different, our behavior is off, we feel destructive to ourselves and to others.

How do we clear these destructive patterns and behaviors and cultivate a consciousness that is strong and steady?

Clearing these patterns and cultivating new ones are benefits of a regular practice of Kundalini Yoga as taught by Yogi Bhajan®. We awaken our intuitive mind and draw upon our deep intelligence and rewrite our destiny on a cellular level. Through our practice we develop the patience to recognize our past, appreciate it for the gifts it delivered, bless it—and then drop it! What a liberating moment in our lives!

As yogis we also acknowledge that we often need help along the way. We turn to different healers, psychologists or spiritual teachers to guide us. They can assist us tremendously by shining a light on our hidden agendas and the problems we face. But it is we who must create the solution and make the changes in our lives. Using the power of prayer, commitment and alignment with the soul and self, we access the vastness of time and space and the Infinite to guide our way forward.

Looking outside of ourselves for the answers will never solve the problem. We have such an incredible gift as women to know the Unknown and see the Unseen. Trust your gift and let go of your insecurity. The greatest downfall of woman is to say: "I don't know." We do know. We were created in the image of the Infinite, and we are the center or nucleus of all creativity. There is nothing lacking in our being.

EACH OF THE KRIYAS AND MEDITATIONS in the following two chapters bring a very powerful healing and lifting of the weight of lifetimes of pain, stress and self-defeating patterns. To let go of our inner anger is to release any imagined disabilities we have created.

Pittra Kriya gives you the blessing of letting go of deep-seated stress and then balances all the chakras.

The **Thunderbolt of Shiva Kriya** cuts through any obstacle in life and clears father phobias.

To clear away old patterns of grief and fear, practice the **Clearing Haunting Thoughts** meditation. A broken heart will never carry us forward in our light and radiance.

Heal this pain and practice the 18th Pauri of *Japji* to release deep feelings of inferiority and self-destructive patterns.

Sahibi Kriya to Master Your Domain and **The Women's Set** both bring incredible strength and resilience to the Self. Make them part of your sadhana routine on a regular basis. **Creating Self-Love** is essential to cultivating a positive relationship to the self—as is opening the heart and making yourself available to receive love. Both of these meditations are powerful, transformative kriyas—one is quiet and contemplative, and the other is a vigorous, almost shocking experience—10,000 volts!

The **Meditation to Strengthen the Inner Voice** cultivates a woman's Fifth Chakra and trust in her intuition. The affirmation practice plants the seed of your true nature and uses the power of *japa* to confirm and reaffirm your Self through your own sound current, your own voice.

Finally, we've included **Sampuran Kriya**, the **33rd Pauri of Japji**, so that you have a technology that opens the gate to the infinite creative flow of the universe, providing a mirror for your own consciousness and creative capacity, and allowing for such a surrender that only the whole of God can fill the space. That's creative longing—that's the key to cultivating the True Self.

PRITPAL KAUR KHALSA
ESPAÑOLA, NEW MEXICO

KRIYA FOR RELIEVING INNER ANGER

SEPTEMBER 21, 1988

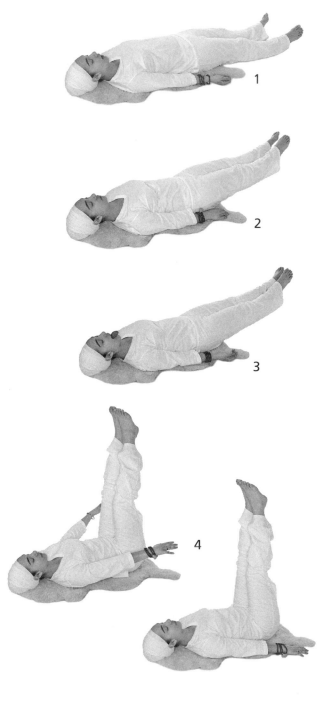

1. Lie down flat on the back in a relaxed posture with arms at the sides, palms open and legs slightly apart. Pretend to snore for **1 1/2 minutes**.

2. Still lying on the back, straighten the legs, point the toes and raise them both up to 6 inches. Hold for **2 minutes**.
This exercise balances anger. It puts pressure on the Navel Point in order to balance the entire system.

3. Remaining in the posture, stick out the tongue and do Breath of Fire through the mouth for **1 1/2 minutes**.

4. Still on the back, lift the legs up to 90 degrees. Keep the arms on the ground by your sides. Begin to beat the ground with all the anger you can achieve. Beat hard and fast for **2 1/2 minutes**, keeping the arms stiff and straight.

5. Still on the back, bring the knees into the chest, and stick the tongue out. Inhale through the open mouth and exhale through the nose. Continue for **3 minutes**.

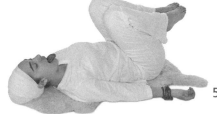

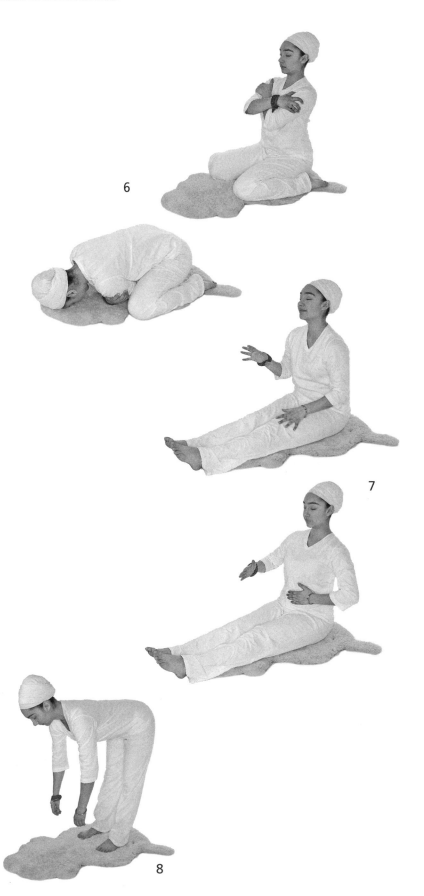

6. Sit in **Celibate Pose**, buttocks on the floor between the heels. Cross the arms over the chest and press them hard against the rib cage. Bend forward and touch the forehead to the floor as if you are bowing. For **2 1/2 minutes** move at a pace of approximately **30 bows per minute**, then for another **30 seconds** speed up and move as fast as you can.

7. Sitting with the legs straight out in front, begin to beat all parts of your body with open palms. Move fast for **2 minutes**.

8. Stand up. Bend forward, keeping the back parallel to the ground, and let the arms and hands hang loose. Remain in this posture and sing for **3 minutes**. (In class, Yogi Bhajan played a recording of *Guru Guru Wahe Guru, Guru Ram Das Guru*.)

9. Continue singing and come into **Cobra Pose**:
Lying on the stomach, place hands under the shoulders
with palms flat. Elongate the spine, lift the chest and
heart up, drop the shoulders, and stretch the head back.
Straighten the arms. Continue for **1 minute**.
Begin circling the neck and continue to sing for another
30 seconds.

10. Still in **Cobra Pose** begin kicking the ground with
alternate feet for **30 seconds**.

11. **Sat Kriya in Easy Pose**. Sit in Easy Pose and close
the eyes. Stretch the arms overhead, keeping the elbows straight. Interlace the fingers with the Jupiter
(index) fingers extended and pointing straight up.
Squeeze the Navel Point in and up as you say "*sat
(sut)*." Release as you chant "*naam*." Continue for **3
minutes**. To end, inhale and squeeze the muscles tightly from the buttocks all the way up the back. Mentally
allow the energy to flow through the top of the skull.
Exhale and relax.

12. **Relaxation**. Lie down and nap on your back for **5
minutes**.

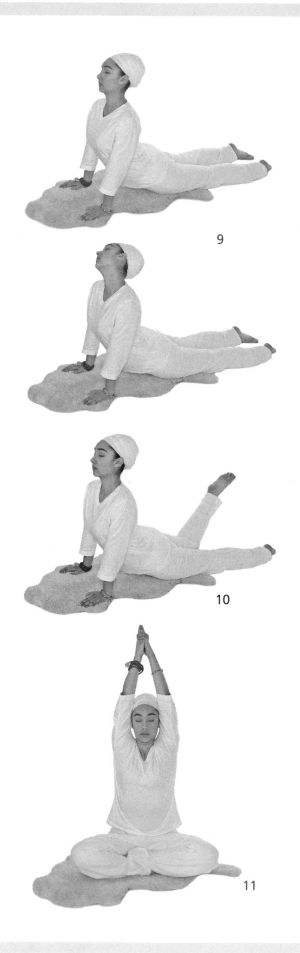

9

10

11

PITTRA KRIYA

NOVEMBER 18, 1991

1. The left hand rests on the Heart Center, right hand cupped in front of you, with the elbow relaxed by your side. Eyes are focused on the tip of the nose. The right hand lifts up and passes the ear, as if you are splashing water over your shoulder. Feel the wind pass the ear as the hand moves toward the shoulder. The wrist must cross the earlobe; the hand must travel that far back. **11 minutes**.

TO END: Inhale, stretch the hand back as far as you can, and suspend the breath for **15 seconds**. Exhale. Repeat two more times.

"It will hit the kidney energy, start working with the adrenals, and then the whole system—the lungs, the central line, your hip-area, pelvic bone area. It is going to affect your body and you will become very relaxed. Do it with a rhythm and do it with a devotion and do it just to get rid of this stress. Get rid of this inner mental and physical tension. You are your vitality. Minus tension, you are fine." — Yogi Bhajan

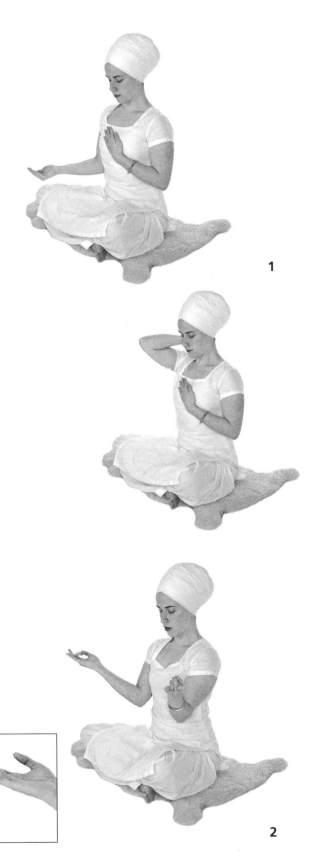

1

2. Place the elbows on the second rib below the base of the breast, in line with the nipple. Hands are slightly wider than the elbows and the palms are facing up in Shuni Mudra. The thumb covers the nail of the Saturn (middle) finger. Eyes are focused at the tip of the nose. As you repeat *HAR*, flick the Saturn finger. The sound *HAR* is very specific and made with the tip of the tongue. The mouth remains slightly open as you generate the sound. **11 minutes**.

TO END: Inhale deeply. Continue moving the fingers. Suspend the breath for **15 seconds**. Let it open the ribcage. It will balance the chakras. Cannon Fire exhale. Repeat three more times.

You have to touch the upper palate—34, 35, 36 meridian points that relate to the hypothalamus will regulate the pituitary and take the secretion which you have created and start asking the energy to open up the chakra. It will start changing the serum of your spine. It will revitalize the gray matter in the brain.

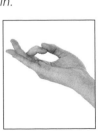

SHUNI MUDRA

2

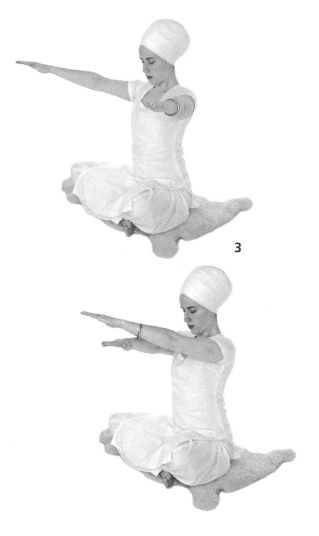

3

3. Bring the arms out in front of you in a V, about 15° above shoulder height. Superman Pose. Hands are flat and facing down. At the rate of one repetition per second, repeat *HAR* as in the second exercise, crossing the hands in front of you and keeping the arms straight. Do not bend the elbows. Alternately cross one hand over the other. Eyes are at the tip of the nose. **11 minutes.**

TO END: Keep moving the arms and inhale, hold for **10 seconds** and Cannon Breath out. Repeat three more times, moving the hands as fast as possible during the last repetition.

These kriyas must be done together and should never be done for ***less than or more than*** 11 minutes each.

About This Kriya

"If you can spare 33 minutes in your life to do this kriya, you can eat up your own stress. The first exercise is going to take care of your glandular system and will affect the liver; it will relax you. The second exercise will balance the chakras. The third exercise will balance your parasympathetic and sympathetic nervous systems." — Yogi Bhajan

This kriya is fantastic for releasing stress. It has a long history in India. When people were filled with grief over the death of a loved one or a tragedy of some sort, they did this first exercise standing in a river. Rivers were seen as the flow of life, as sacred and healing. They would toss the water over their shoulder. The yogis knew that the brain had to be restarted, broken out of the frozen state that stress produces.

This kriya works best if practiced regularly for a while. Yogi Bhajan explained that many people would do it a few times but then stop before the full benefit ripened; they would not do a full 40-day *sadhana*. So the priests connected the practice to *Surya Namaskar*, or worshipping the source of life, the sun, the inner spirit. This element of worship made it a more meaningful practice to them, more than just an effective technology of self-stimulation and self-adjustment. But, in fact, if you do this practice without a river and without belief in anything but your own Infinite Self, it works wonders.

Yogi Bhajan asked us to share this kriya, to give it to our friends, family, students and strangers, too. He said that it would save a lot of trouble in life. *"Once you restore your own vitality, you can enjoy your virtues."*

STRESS RELIEF AND CLEARING THE EMOTIONS OF THE PAST

NOVEMBER 18, 1991

POSTURE: Sit in Easy Pose with a straight spine.

MUDRA: Place the hands at the center of the chest with the tips of the thumbs touching each other and each of the fingers touching the corresponding fingers on the opposite hand. Leave space between the palms. The fingertips are pointing upward.

EYE FOCUS: Look at the tip of the nose.

BREATH PATTERN: Breathe 4 times per minute: inhale 5 seconds, hold 5 seconds, exhale 5 seconds.

TIME: Continue for **11 minutes** or until you feel relief from the stress.

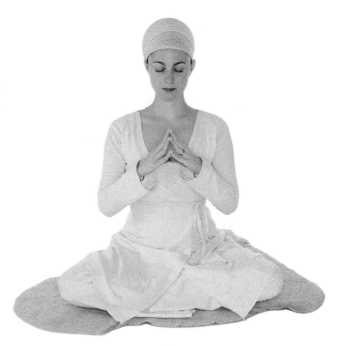

About This Meditation

This meditation is especially useful for dealing with stressful relationships and with past family issues. It addresses phobias, fears, and neuroses. It can remove unsettling thoughts from the past that surface into the present. It can take difficult situations in the present and release them into the Hands of Infinity.

TERSHULA KRIYA
THUNDERBOLT OF SHIVA

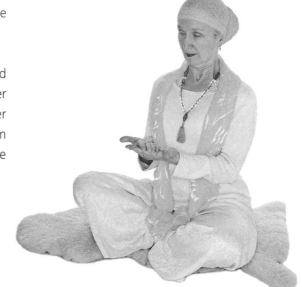

POSTURE: Sit in Easy Pose with a straight spine, and a light Neck Lock.

EYE FOCUS: The eyes are closed, and looking at the back of the eyelids.

MUDRA: Bring the elbows next to the ribs, forearms extended in front of you, with the hands in front of the heart, right over left, palms up. The hands are approximately 10 degrees higher than the elbows. There is no bend in the wrists. The arms from the fingertips to the elbows form a straight line. The thumbs are extended out to the sides of the hands.

MANTRA: Mentally chant the mantra *Har Har Wahe Guru*:

HAR HAR WHAA-HAY GUROO

BREATH & VISUALIZATION: Inhale through the nostrils, pull back on the navel, and suspend the breath. Mentally chant the mantra for as long as you are able to retain the breath. While chanting, visualize your hands surrounded by white light. Exhale through the nostrils and visualize lightning shooting out from your fingertips. When you have completely exhaled, hold the breath out, pull *mulbandh*, and again mentally recite the mantra as long as you are able. Inhale deeply and continue.

TIME: 31-62 minutes.

About This Meditation

Tershula is the thunderbolt of Shiva, one of the Hindu Trinity of gods: Brahma, Vishnu and Shiva. Shiva is the destroyer or regenerator. *Tershula* can activate the self-healing process. This meditation balances the three *gunas*—the three qualities that permeate all creation: *rajas, tamas,* and *sattva*. It brings the three nervous systems together. It gives you the ability to heal at a distance, through your touch or through your projection. Many psychological disorders or imbalances in the personality can be cured through practice of this kriya. It is helpful in getting rid of phobias, especially father phobia.

It is suggested that this meditation be done in a cool room, or at night when the temperature is cooler, because it directly stimulates the kundalini and generates a great deal of heat in the body.

KRIYA TO REMOVE HAUNTING THOUGHTS
TEN STEPS TO PEACE

POSTURE: Sit comfortably.

EYE FOCUS: Lower the eyelids until the eyes are only open 1/10th. Concentrate on the tip of the nose.

MANTRA: In this Ten Step process, you will be silently, mentally chanting *Wahe Guru* in the following manner:

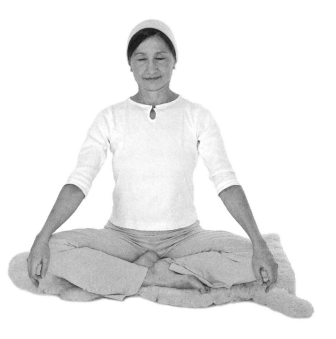

WHAA	Mentally focus on the right eye.
HAY	Mentally focus on the left eye.
GUROO	Mentally focus on the tip of the nose.

One   Inhale, exhale and mentally say *WAHE GURU.*

Two   Inhale and bring to mind the encounter or incident which happened to you.

Three   Exhale and mentally say *WAHE GURU*.

Four   Inhale. Visualize and relive the actual feeling of the encounter.

Five   Exhale and again mentally repeat *WAHE GURU*.

Six   Inhale and reverse roles in the encounter you are remembering. Become the other person and experience their perspective.

Seven   Exhale and mentally repeat *WAHE GURU*.

Eight   Inhale. Forgive the other person and forgive yourself.

Nine   Exhale and mentally repeat *WAHE GURU*.

Ten   Inhale. Let go of the incident and release it into the Universe.

MEDITATION TO HEAL A BROKEN HEART

MARCH 26, 1975

POSTURE: Sit in Easy Pose with a straight spine, and a light Neck Lock.

MUDRA: Palms together, lightly touching. The tip of the Saturn (middle) finger is at the level of the Third Eye Point. The forearms are horizontal to the ground, elbows high. Look within.

(No mantra or breath specified.)

TIME: Continue for **11, 31 or 62 minutes**.

TO END: Inhale, exhale, relax the breath, and with clasped hands stretch the arms up for **2 minutes**.

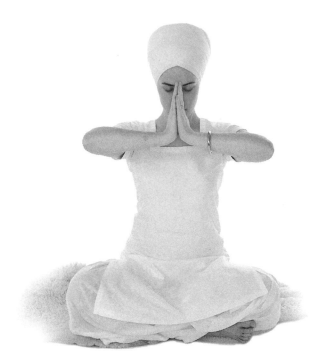

About This Meditation

This meditation is very relaxing if you understand it. The autonomic system will relax and your breath will automatically move toward a meditative pace to renew and relax your heart and mind.

To heal the emotional wounds of the heart we need to bring calm to the nerves that hold the wound. We know that a break in relationship (to others or to our Self) has almost identical reactions in the nervous system and brain as a physical injury or loss of limb.

This mudra creates balance; it generates a subtle pressure which adjusts the heart meridian along the little finger and outer forearm, activating the "action nerve" junction with the autonomic system to reset itself by keeping the forearms parallel to the ground and involving the armpit reflexes; and finally, it uses the pranic influence of the middle finger and its Saturn and air qualities to quell residual emotional storms.

MAKING PEACE WITH THE SHADOW
THE 18TH PAURI OF JAPJI SAHIB

Shabd Guru

MAKING PEACE WITH THE SHADOW SIDE OF LIFE can be very difficult. For most of us, we have been given a vision of life, and the universe, where the power of the Light is considered Divine and the power of Darkness is considered something else. This creates a duality within us, which refuses to acknowledge the shadow in ourselves, and judges and reacts to the shadow in other people.

Guru Nanak gives a different understanding. In the 18th Pauri of *Japji Sahib*, Guru Nanak describes the darkest, most shadowed aspects of the human personality—and then, in humility, acknowledges that all this shadow is also part of the divine. The Creator created it. It has a purpose. A purpose that is often beyond the understanding of our limited human mind, but is totally understandable from the perspective of the One who forms, organizes and governs the entire creation. The shadow has a reason for existing; the shadow within us and within others has a definite purpose and power; it is part of *hukam*—the divine order of the universe. It is the challenge through which we grow. It is the pain which brings us to even deeper levels of healing. The shadow forces us to face what we do not want to face, and make peace with what we do not want to acknowledge.

The point of a spiritual practice is not to get rid of the shadow. In fact, it's not even possible to get rid of it. Instead, the point of spiritual practice is to become aware of the shadow, to bring it out into the light, so that it does not take over your life. Yogi Bhajan would sometimes say, "The only difference between me and other people is that I am aware of my weaknesses." Weaknesses exist. When we are blind to them, they create havoc in our lives. When we are aware of them, then we can restrain them, and consciously work with them to understand their purpose and gift.

In the last lines of the 18th *Pauri*, Guru Nanak claims, "What pleases Thee is the only good worth doing." It is a humble acknowledgement that while we may not like the shadow side of life, if it pleases the Creator for the shadow to exist, then there is something good in it. In that state of humility, we can heal our own fractured sense of self. Rather than dividing ourselves into our "good parts" and "bad parts," we can embrace all aspects as given to us by the Creator, and know that they all have a purpose. This restores us to a holistic vision of life—and it is in this holistic vision that ultimately we find peace, ease and happiness.

Suggestions for Practice

Recite the 18th Pauri 11 times a day for 40 day, 90 days, 120 days or 1,000 days to clear yourself of attachment to good and bad, to overcome deep feelings of inferiority, to break self-destructive behavior patterns and to surrender in complete acceptance of what is—both in yourself and in others.

EK ONG KAAR KAUR KHALSA
ESPAÑOLA, NEW MEXICO

ਆਸੰਖ ਮੂਰਖ ਅੰਧ ਘੋਰ ਆਸੰਖ ਚੋਰ ਹਰਾਮਖੋਰ

MAKING PEACE WITH THE SHADOW
THE 18TH PAURI OF JAPJI SAHIB

ਅਸੰਖ ਮੂਰਖ ਅੰਧ ਘੋਰ ॥ ਅਸੰਖ ਚੋਰ ਹਰਾਮਖੋਰ ॥
ਅਸੰਖ ਅਮਰ ਕਰਿ ਜਾਹਿ ਜੋਰ ॥ ਅਸੰਖ ਗਲਵਢ ਹਤਿਆ ਕਮਾਹਿ ॥
ਅਸੰਖ ਪਾਪੀ ਪਾਪੁ ਕਰਿ ਜਾਹਿ ॥ ਅਸੰਖ ਕੂੜਿਆਰ ਕੂੜੇ ਫਿਰਾਹਿ ॥
ਅਸੰਖ ਮਲੇਛ ਮਲੁ ਭਖਿ ਖਾਹਿ ॥ ਅਸੰਖ ਨਿੰਦਕ ਸਿਰਿ ਕਰਹਿ ਭਾਰੁ ॥
ਨਾਨਕੁ ਨੀਚੁ ਕਹੈ ਵਿਚਾਰੁ ॥ ਵਾਰਿਆ ਨ ਜਾਵਾ ਏਕ ਵਾਰ ॥
ਜੋ ਤੁਧੁ ਭਾਵੈ ਸਾਈ ਭਲੀ ਕਾਰ ॥ ਤੂ ਸਦਾ ਸਲਾਮਤਿ ਨਿਰੰਕਾਰ ॥੧੮॥

Asankh moorakh andh ghor. Asankh chor haraamkhor.
Asankh amar kar jaahi jor. Asankh galvadh hati-aa kamaahi.
Asankh paapee paap kar jaahi. Asankh koorhi-aar koorhay firaahi.
Asankh malaychh mal bhakh khaahi. Asankh nindak sir karahi bhaar.
Naanak neech kahai veechaar. Vaari-aa na jaavaa ayk vaar.
Jo tudh bhaavai saa-ee bhalee kaar. Too sadaa salaamat nirankaar. 18

Countless fools, blinded by ignorance. Countless thieves and cheaters.
Countless impose their will by force. Countless cut-throats gather sins.
Countless sinners who keep on sinning. Countless liars, wander lost in their lies.
Countless wretches, eat filth for food. Countless slanders, make their heads heavy
Lowly Nanak, gives this explanation. I cannot even begin to describe You.
Whatever pleases You, All will be blessed, You always protect us, Formless One! 18

Woman as Her Own Psychologist II

CULTIVATING THE SELF

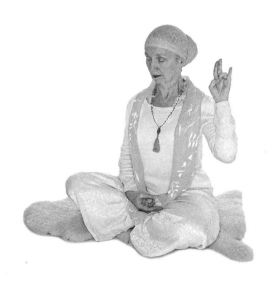

LOOKING OUTSIDE OF OURSELVES for the answers will never solve the problem. We have such an incredible gift as women to know the Unknown and see the Unseen. Trust your gift and let go of your insecurity.

THE WOMAN'S SET

1. **Rock Pose**. Sit on heels, palms on thighs or hands relaxed on lap, spine straight. Relax meditatively in this position. **3 minutes**

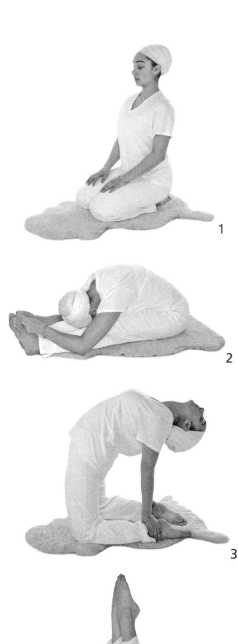

2. **Life Nerve Stretch**. For this set, Life Nerve Stretch can be done in 3 ways:

  (a) Sit on the right heel, left leg extended straight out.
      Change sides. **3 minutes on each side**.

  Or

  (b) Extend the left leg straight, and draw the right foot to groin.
      Change sides. **3 minutes on each side**.

  Or

  (c) Extend both legs straight out in front. **3 minutes**.

Grab the big toe(s) in finger-lock. Inhale, lengthen the spine. Exhale, bend forward bringing chest to thighs, and nose to knees. Avoid leading with the head. In all 3 variations, use Long Deep Breathing.

3. **Camel Pose**. Come up onto the knees, thighs perpendicular to the floor. Arch back, holding onto heels. Let head fall back, press hips forward. Long, deep breathing. **3 minutes**. *This exercise adjusts the reproductive organs.*

4. **Shoulder Stand**. From lying on the back, place the hands on the hips, just below the waist, and bring the hips and legs up to a vertical position, spine and legs perpendicular to the ground. Support the weight of the body on the elbows and shoulders using the hands to support the lower spine. The chin is pressed into the chest. Long, deep breathing. **3 minutes**
This exercise releases pressure on all of the organs and stimulates the thyroid gland.

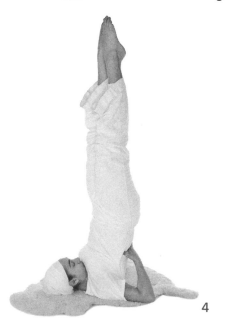

5. **Archer Pose**. Bring the right foot forward so that the feet are 2-3 feet apart. The right toes face forward while the left foot comes to a 45 degree angle, with the heel back and the toes forward. The left leg stays straight and strong as the right knee bends until the thigh is almost parallel to the ground (do not let the knee go beyond the toes); tuck the tailbone. Curl the fingers of both hands onto the palms, thumbs pulled back. As if pulling back a bow and arrow, lift the right arm up, extended forward parallel to the ground, over the right knee. The left arm, bent at the elbow, pulls back until the fist is at the left shoulder. Pull Neck Lock. Chin in, chest out. Feel this stretch across the chest. Eyes stare beyond the thumb to Infinity. Practice for **5 minutes on each side**.

6. **Baby Pose**. Sit on the heels. Bring the forehead to ground. Arms relaxed at the sides with palms facing up. **3 minutes**.

7. **Bow Pose**. Come onto the stomach. Grab the ankles, and use the thigh muscles to pull the upper body off the ground. Raise the legs off the ground. As the chest lifts, let the head follow. Hold position with Long Deep Breathing. **3 minutes**.

8. **Locust Pose**. Still on the stomach, feet together, with the chin on the ground. Place the fists under the hips where the hips and thighs join. Raise the legs up, and the back of the thighs to keep the legs together. Breathe long and deep. **3 minutes**.

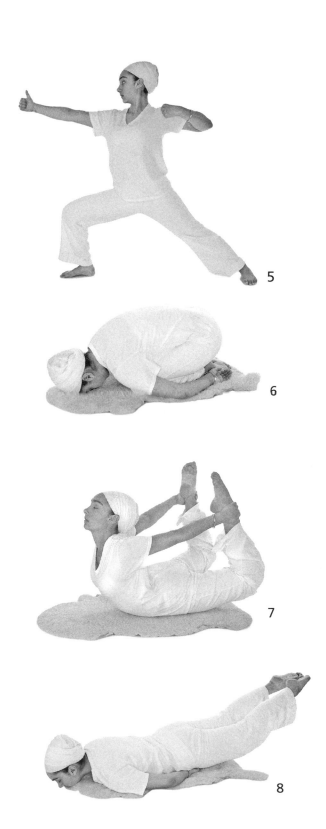

5

6

7

8

9. **Cow Pose**. Come onto the hands and knees. The hands are shoulder-width apart, with fingers facing forward, knees directly under the hips, and the big toes together behind you. Inhale and tilt the pelvis forward, arching the spine down, with head and neck stretched back. Do not scrunch the neck. Open the heart and raise the chin as far as you can without collapsing the neck. Hold with long, deep breathing. **3 minutes.**

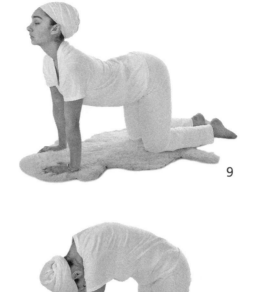

9

10. **Cat Pose**. Beginning in Cow Pose, tilt the pelvis the opposite way, arching the spine up, pressing the chin into the chest, arched up like an angry cat. Hold with long, deep breathing. **3 minutes.**

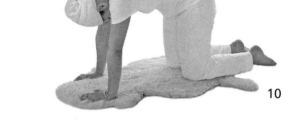

10

11. **Stretch Pose**. Lie on the back with the feet together, toes pointed. Flatten the lower back. Place hands palms down over the thighs, pointing toward the toes. Lift the head up, apply Neck Lock and look at the toes. Lift the feet up 6 inches and begin Breath of Fire for **3 minutes.**

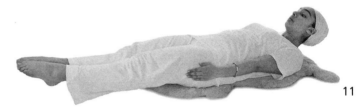

11

12. **Corpse Pose**. Relax on the back, palms facing up. **8-10 minutes.**

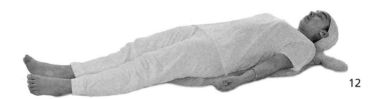

12

About This Kriya

The kriya will take 45 minutes to complete, when practiced for designated times. This kriya is designed to keep your spine, organs and nervous system strong and healthy. It works on keeping the female organs healthy, particularly relieving tension in the ovaries. If practiced everyday it can give you beauty, radiance and grace.

SAHIBI KRIYA TO MASTER YOUR DOMAIN

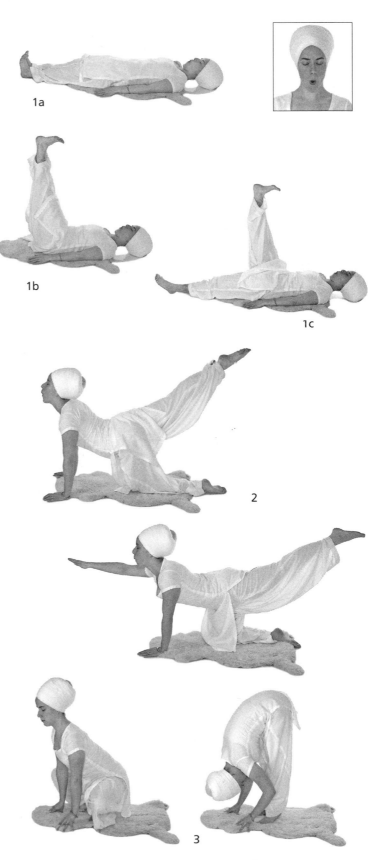

1. Lie on the back with the feet together. Flex the feet toward the head

   (a) Make a firm circle of the mouth and begin Breath of Fire through the mouth.

   (b) Continuing with Breath of Fire, raise the legs straight up to 90 degrees and lower them to the ground keeping the feet and toes flexed and the knees straight. Move rhythmically with the breath for **5 minutes**. Inhale and hold the legs up briefly. Slowly lower the legs to the ground as you exhale.

   (c) Resume the exercise raising alternate legs to 90 degrees. Breathing in the same manner move rapidly for **2 minutes**.

   This exercise helps to correct menstrual irregularities.

2. This is a two-part exercise done in **Cow Pose**.

   (a) First extend alternate legs up and back as high as possible. Begin Breath of Fire through the circled mouth raising and lowering the legs rapidly in rhythm with the breath. Continue for **4 minutes**.

   (b) Remain on the hands and knees. As you raise the right leg up and back, simultaneously extend the left arm straight out in front of the body. Lower them and raise the opposite arm and leg. Continue alternating the arms and legs, moving rhythmically with Breath of Fire through the circled mouth for **2 minutes**. Inhale, exhale, and relax onto the heels.

3. Come into **Frog Pose**. Squat down on the toes, knees wide apart. Heels are touching, and raised up off the ground. Place the fingertips on the ground between the knees. The face is forward. Inhale as you raise the hips up, keeping the fingertips on the ground, heels up, knees locked. Exhale down, face forward, knees outside of arms. Continue moving rhythmically and rapidly **52 times**.

4. Sit in Easy Pose with the navel pulled in and chest out. Tuck the chin in to form a straight line from the base of the spine to the top of the head and lock yourself in this posture. Extend your arms up to 60 degrees with the palms facing each other. Keep the arms straight with no bend in the elbows. Inhale and extend the arms up to 90 degrees, then exhale and lower the arms to 60 degrees Continue for **5 minutes** taking one complete breath every 2 seconds. *(The recording of Jaap Sahib by Ragi Sat Nam Singh is used.)* Extend the arms straight up to 90 degrees on the first accented beat—*Namastang* or *Namo*, then back down to 60° on the second beat. Do not move at all during musical phrases. Do this as a perfect drill through Verse 28 *(to Chaachree Chand)*. Move in perfect rhythm with the music. To end, inhale, exhale and relax.

Physically this exercise stimulates the heart, circulatory system and glandular system. It works powerfully on the mental realm as well, training you to concentrate and gain control of your mind and 'sahibi' or control over your domain.

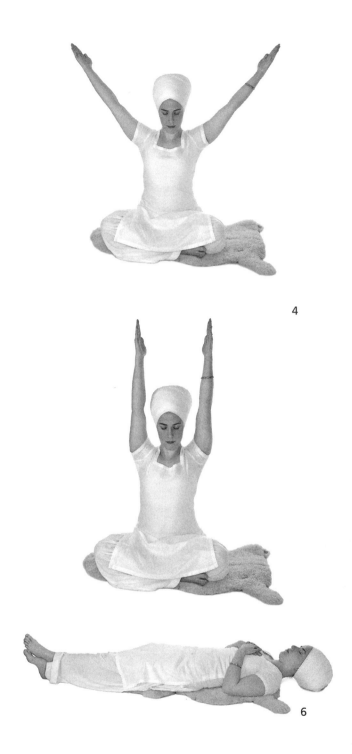

4

5. Remain in Easy Pose. Breathe long and deep and meditate to the music for **5 minutes**. *(The song Himalaya by Sat Peter Singh was played in the original class. Select any uplifting and relaxing 3HO music.)*

6. Lie down on the back with the legs crossed at the ankles and hands crossed over the heart. Relax in this position and breathe long and deep for **5 minutes**. *(The song Promises by Sat Peter Singh was played in the original class. Select any uplifting and relaxing 3HO music and relax.)*

6

About This Kriya

When you control your domain you act from the center of your being. In the realm of mind it means you can hold and project an important thought. In the realm of body it means you are able to circulate blood from the core to the outlying limbs and glands. This kriya gives you that command in both realms.

The deep muscular tension released through these exercises enables the blood to flow freely to all parts of the body, feeding the cells with oxygen and nutrients, and flushing the body of toxins and the byproducts of normal metabolism.

CREATING SELF-LOVE

APRIL 4, 1994

1. Sit in Easy Pose with a straight spine. Hold the right palm six to nine inches above the top center of the head. The right palm faces down, blessing you. This self-blessing corrects the aura. The left elbow is bent with the upper arm near the rib cage. The left palm faces forward and blesses the world. The eyes are closed and focus at the lunar center in the middle of the chin. Breathe long, slow and deep with a feeling of self-affection. Try to breathe only **one breath per minute**: **Inhale 20 seconds, hold 20 seconds, exhale 20 seconds. 11 minutes**. Inhale deeply and move slowly and directly into position for exercise two.

2. Extend the arms straight out in front, parallel to the ground, palms facing down. Stretch out to your maximum. The eyes are focused at the lunar center in the center of the chin, and the breath is long, slow and deep. **3 minutes**. Inhale deeply and move slowly and directly into position for exercise three.

3. Stretch the arms straight up with the palms facing forward. There is no bend in the elbows. The eyes are focused at the lunar center and the breath continues to be long, slow and deep. **3 minutes**. To end: Inhale, hold the breath for 10 seconds while you stretch the arms upward (try to stretch so much that your buttocks are lifted) and tighten all the muscles of the body. Exhale. Repeat this sequence two more times.

About This Kriya

The first exercise is called *Reverse Adi Shakti Kriya* in which you are mentally and hypnotically blessing yourself. This self-blessing affects and corrects the magnetic field. Doing this exercise will hurt if you are an angry person. Self-help is very difficult for those who are angry. After doing this exercise for 5 minutes your muscles will also start hurting if your diet is improper. The taste in your mouth will change if you are breathing correctly.

The second exercise will benefit everything between the neck and navel. It will give strength to the heart and will open up the Heart Center.

"Love doesn't rule you. What rules you is fear, phenomenal fear. Through this kriya, love can be invoked and fear can be reduced." — Yogi Bhajan

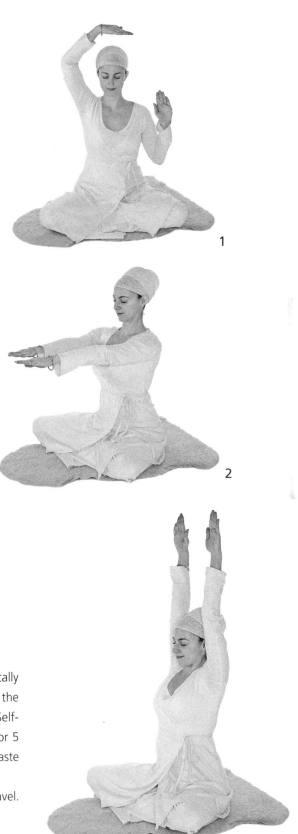

MEDITATION TO OPEN THE LOCK OF THE HEART AND INCREASE THE POWER OF THE INFINITE WITHIN

POSTURE: Sit in Easy Pose with a straight spine, and a light Neck Lock.

MUDRA & MOVEMENT: Bring hands approximately 6-8 inches in front of your face, palms flat and facing one another, fingers pointing toward the ceiling, and with approximately a 6-8 inch space between the palms. Elbows are relaxed down. With a very fast, powerful jerk, stretch the hands out until there is about 36 inches between the hands, and abruptly stop them. Then instantly the hands recoil back to the first position in front of the body. The stopping process will be so abrupt, done with such a powerful force, that you'll find the hands, chest, shoulders, and head jerking back and forth a little bit.

MANTRA: Use the rhythm of the recording *Tantric Har*, or 1 movement per second. Do not sing aloud. On every **HAR**, stretch the arms with such a powerful force, just as if eleven hundred volts have hit you. Concentrate on the reaction in your chest.

EYE FOCUS: Unspecified.

TIME: 11 minutes.

END: Inhale and suspend the breath, but keep on doing the motion on the held breath for approximately 15 seconds. Exhale. Inhale again and continue the motion for approximately 10 seconds. Exhale. Inhale deeply, continue, holding for approximately 5 seconds. Relax.

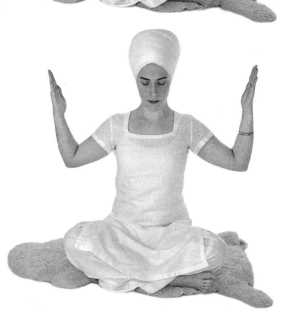

About This Meditation

The chest area is called the Heart Chakra. This heavy jolt, as you spring your hands and arms apart, will cause a jerking reaction to your chest cavity, which will open up your Heart Center. Opening of your Heart Center cavity is opening up to your own Infinity. The navel area, the Third Chakra, is sometimes referred to as the *agan granthi*—the place from which all fire-related activites spring—food, digestion, breath, to name a few. When this center is locked, your ribcage can become out of place. Then the diaphragm doesn't act right, and you lose one third of your life force. This meditation releases this lock and will open up the power of the Almighty within you. You must bring forth the entire power of your being, using a great force with the movement. In this way you will shock your subtle nervous system on the sound of *Har*. Through this meditation you can move the power of the *ida* and *pingala*, and open up the *sushmuna*.

MEDITATION TO STRENGTHEN THE INNER VOICE

PART ONE

POSTURE: Sit with a straight spine in Easy Pose or Lotus Pose.

MUDRA & BREATH PATTERN: Cup the hands lightly together. Leave a slit between the outer sides of the little fingers. Bow the head forward over the palms. Look into the palms, eyes barely open. Inhale in **10 strokes**, mentally vibrating *WHAA-HO* with each stroke. Exhale in **10 strokes**, each time mentally vibrating *GUROO*.

TIME: Continue for **11 minutes**. Then inhale powerfully, exhale powerfully, and relax.

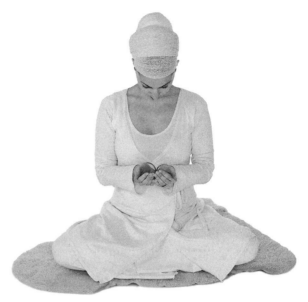

PART TWO

Still sitting in Easy Pose, hands in Gyan Mudra, chant in a continuous monotone:

WHAA-HO WHAA-HO WHAA-HO WHAA-HO
WHAA-HO WHAA-HO WHAA-HO WHAA-HO
GUROO GUROO GUROO GUROO
GUROO GUROO GUROO GUROO

TIME: Continue for **5-11 minutes**. You may build up to 31 minutes on this meditation.

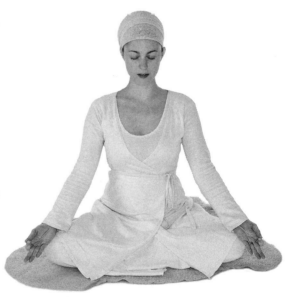

About This Meditation

At times when the path of truth and clarity seems lost, calm yourself and still your mind. Then the path will be shown to you. In this meditation the head is bent as if in offering to the Guru or the Higher Self. Besides strengthening your mental direction, it can alleviate any blood disease. To live life according to the guidance of inner truth is essential. If you do not, you will have doubts. If doubts are not removed, then frustration comes in. Frustration, when not released, leads to anger. Anger then leads to destructive action either to the Self, others, or both. To stop this vicious cycle, create the habit to still the Self and ask questions of your own higher consciousness. This meditation can develop that capacity.

"Watch out for your worst enemy —that is whosoever steals your stability is your worst enemy. It's not evil—that makes you strong. Rather it is those who lay emotional tantrums. They say, "You are no friend if you are not miserable when I am." We must work together against our own sickness."   — Yogi Bhajan

I AM A WOMAN: AFFIRMATION PRACTICE

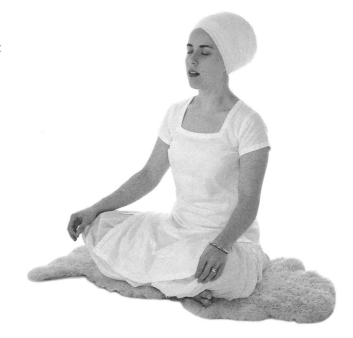

POSTURE: Sit comfortably and recite these affirmations:

> *GOD MADE ME A WOMAN.*
> *I AM A WOMAN TO BE.*
> *NOW NOW NOW.*

TIME: 3-31 minutes.

About These Affirmations

"These are the strongest affirmations you can ever utter. The moment you make the tongue rotate, watch the tip of the upper palate stimulate your entire psyche and force the neurons to adjust their balance right there—on the spot. The hypothalmus immediately communicates with the subconscious memory to release your strength and all the strength of every woman grand, grand, great, great, great, super—two million generations from which your egg has come through, and confront the spermatazoa." —Yogi Bhajan

God made me a woman

The infinity. Woman contains the man in it. God is responsible for making it. You do not take the blame. This gets rid of the blame. You recognize your ego to be God's Will. Nobody can get rid of ego, but you can convert your ego into God's Will.

I am a woman to be

This is an affirmation of your own honour, nobility, self-love, creativity, to get rid of the crisis and conflict that are within you.

Now Now Now

It is the elevating power to face the now. Capture and elevate yourself above time. You say three times: "In the past I have done it. I am going to do it. I am going to do it no matter what."

SAMPURAN KRIYA
THE 33RD PAURI OF JAPJI SAHIB

Shabd Guru

"Whosoever chants the 33rd pauri of Japji Sahib 25 times a day, there is nothing on Earth he will not have. Guru Nanak sang this pauri as a sampuran kriya, a perfect, perfect seal. This pauri means that if you ask for nothing, you will get everything—that is the law. Whosoever chants this pauri 25 times a day, there is nothing on the Earth that he or she will not have. Ask for nothing, just praise the Lord."

—Yogi Bhajan, July 3, 1982

Sometimes as humans we forget that the One who created us really does love us. We spend our lives looking for a sense of security. We search for that security in the material world, rather than searching for it in the love of the Creator. The opposite of love is not hate. The opposite of love is fear. Fear is what kills the experience of love. We do so many things on the material plane in an attempt to prevent fear from taking over our lives. We try to build security for ourselves just to keep fear at bay, hoping that one day, the love we long for will come.

Guru Nanak understood that about human nature. In the 33rd *Pauri* he gives a very effective antidote to fear. All of the things we long for, all that we are worried about, all of our striving, all of the images we create in our minds of what constitutes security, Guru Nanak takes that list and says, "I have no power to do any of this. I have no power to live. I have no power to die. I have no power to accumulate wealth. I have no power to liberate myself. All of that power is in Your Hands, Oh Divine Creator of mine."

For those with children, you know that there are times when you want to help them, but they stubbornly turn away. They may need your help, but they do not want your help. They want to figure it out for themselves—how to do something, how to get something—this is the way we treat the Creator. The Divine created us and has the power to create everything for us. But we turn away, wanting to do it on our own. Like a kind, loving parent, the Divine watches with a smile, and waits patiently for that moment when we will say, "I can't do it. I don't have the power to do it. If it pleases You, You can do it for me."

Suggested Practice

The 33rd *Pauri*, when recited 25 times a day, brings us to that state of surrender, where we realize, Wow, I really can't do it. I really have no power. But there is a Loving Universal Infinite Divine Creator—and the hand of that One can do it all. So let's stop this illusion that we have the power, and let's just appreciate the hand of that One, and what It's already done for us. In such a consciousness, we discover and find that Love is there. Love has been there all along, and by accepting what the Loving Creator wants to bring us, we have all the security we need.

EK ONG KAAR KAUR KHALSA
ESPAÑOLA, NEW MEXICO

ਆਖਹਿ ਜੋਰ ਚੁਪੈ ਨਹ ਜੋਰ ਜੋਰ ਨ ਮੰਗਣਿ ਦੇਇ ਨ ਜੋਰ

SAMPURAN KRIYA
THE 33RD PAURI OF JAPJI SAHIB

ਆਖਣਿ ਜੋਰੁ ਚੁਪੈ ਨਹ ਜੋਰੁ
ਜੋਰੁ ਨ ਮੰਗਣਿ ਦੇਣਿ ਨ ਜੋਰੁ
ਜੋਰੁ ਨ ਜੀਵਣਿ ਮਰਣਿ ਨਹ ਜੋਰੁ
ਜੋਰੁ ਨ ਰਾਜਿ ਮਾਲਿ ਮਨਿ ਸੋਰੁ
ਜੋਰੁ ਨ ਸੁਰਤੀ ਗਿਆਨਿ ਵੀਚਾਰਿ
ਜੋਰੁ ਨ ਜੁਗਤੀ ਛੁਟੈ ਸੰਸਾਰੁ
ਜਿਸੁ ਹਥਿ ਜੋਰੁ ਕਰਿ ਵੇਖੈ ਸੋਇ
ਨਾਨਕ ਉਤਮੁ ਨੀਚੁ ਨ ਕੋਇ ॥੩੩॥

Aakhan jor chupai nah jor. Jor na mangan dayn na jor.
Jor na jeevan maran nah jor. Jor na raaj maal man sor.
Jor na surtee gi-aan veechaar. Jor na jugtee chhutai sansaar.
Jis hath jor kar vaykhai so-ay. Naanak utam neech na ko-ay. 33

Uttering brings power; silence brings no power.
Power is not gained by begging; giving doesn't bring power.
Power is not gained by living; death doesn't bring power.
Power is not gained by ruling with wealth and occult mental powers.
Power is not gained by understanding, spiritual wisdom and meditation.
Power is not gained by finding a way to escape from the world.
In whose Hand the Power is, He watches over all.
O Nanak, no one is high or low. 33

CRISIS KIT

WHAT TO DO WHEN THERE'S NOTHING LEFT TO DO

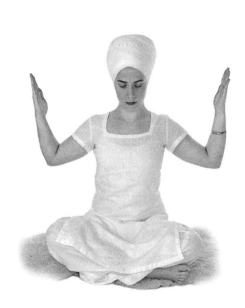

AS WOMEN, we have the infinite capacity to turn emotion into devotion, return to our basic core, engage the calming influence of the breath, and act from intuition rather than impulse.

DURING THE POWERFUL AND TRANSFORMATIVE YEARS of Khalsa Women's Training Camp with Yogi Bhajan, he often stressed the key qualities within the nature of a successful woman—and also those characteristics that trip her up. He would tell stories, share examples, have us sing songs, and invite us to tell our own stories. He would basically employ any method possible to get the message across.

One such message was how, as women, we often make mistakes when we attempt to go out and get what we think we need in our lives. He repeated over and over again that the key to our success was to be still and allow things to come to us. As women, we've been trained to look outside of ourselves to someone or something else for solutions. Yet, it's when we access and deeply listen to the pool of consciousness within that our strength and power as a woman is activated. The truest test of our ability to access our intuition and grace when we most need it is when we are in crisis. These are the times when we are likely to react, become commotional, flip out, freak out, and fall victim to our own skittering mind, desperate for a solution. In that pattern, and within that reality, we solve nothing. We only create more drama. However, as women, we have the infinite capacity to turn emotion into devotion, return to our basic core, engage the calming influence of the breath, and act from intuition rather than impulse.

Suggestions for Practice

The selection of kriyas and meditations offered in this section is a powerful toolkit to draw from to help you return to your center, go inside, and dwell in the subtle pool of self-mastery. Some of the techniques build your long-term capacity to deal with stress and develop the fortitude to hold up under difficulty. Others can be used in the heat of the moment to deal with immediate challenges, alter your energy, and enable you to cope.

With **The Kriya to Throw Off Stress**, you develop your internal strength by fortifying your glandular system, intelligence and consciousness. This provides the internal solidity to be effective.

The **Kriya to Withstand the Pressure of the Time** is an overall tonic for building the nervous system and the capacity to hold up. This kriya gives you the strength to choose excellence at the moment that you need it.

Only five repetitions of the mantra in **The Meditation for Absolutely Powerful Energy** are required to give you the energy to face a difficult day ahead or to deal with 'brain drain'.

The Meditation to Fight Brain Fatigue balances the diaphragm and helps you live to your excellence.

The Meditation to Prevent Freaking Out trains you to alter your energy and calm down when you need it.

In just three minutes of practice, **The Meditation to Neutralize the Mind** can tranquilize the mind and help you find relaxation and peace.

Practicing **The Meditation for the Restless Mind** for just three minutes gives the capacity to still your restlessness and find a moment of equanimity from which to act.

The Triple Mantra clear obstacles and provides protection.

Yogi Bhajan's instruction about **The Last Resort Meditation** is to practice it when life doesn't work for you, and you can't go to anyone about it. It will enable you to think right, act right, see right, look at yourself clearly and meditate.

Everything else will follow.

DEV SUROOP KAUR KHALSA
ESPAÑOLA, NEW MEXICO

KRIYA TO THROW OFF STRESS

JANUARY 24, 1990

1. Sit in Easy Pose with a straight spine. Bring the hands up by your shoulders with the palms forward and the fingers pointing upward. Touch the thumb and the Jupiter (index) finger and then touch the thumb and the Sun (ring) finger. Continue rapidly touching the thumb alternately with each of the two fingers. Concentrate on the tip of your nose. Keep your eyes open. The ideal speed for this action is 9 touches per second, but 3 touches per second is acceptable. After **5-1/2 minutes**, begin inhaling and exhaling powerfully through the mouth. Breathe through the mouth for **2 minutes** and then begin Breath of Fire through the nose for another **30 seconds**. Inhale deeply and relax. *This exercise adjusts the ovaries, stimulates the life force energy, and releases stress.*

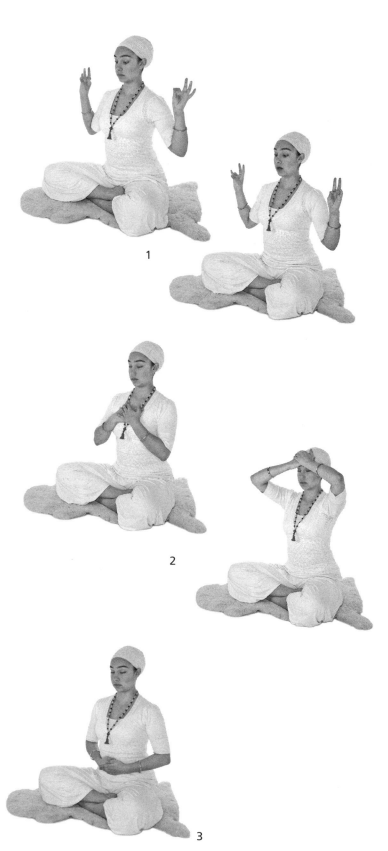

2. (a) Cross the hands over the Heart Center, left hand on top of the right. Close the eyes and breathe extremely deeply and slowly as you feel the healing strength of your own hands on your heart. **4 minutes**.

(b) Put both hands on your forehead, feeling the healing effect of your hands. Concentrate on *"I am, I am"* as you listen to Nirinjan Kaur's *Bountiful, Blissful and Beautiful*. **7 minutes**.

3. Put both hands on the Navel Point and press with all your force. Breathe slowly and meditate deeply on Nirinjan Kaur's *Ong Namo, Guru Dev Namo*. **8 minutes**. Inhale deeply, open your eyes and shake your hands.

4. Twist the wrists back and forth, keeping the five fingers spread open. **2 minutes**.
This is to change the neurons of the brain.

5. Place the hands on the shoulders and sing along with Guru Shabad Singh's recording of *Pavan Pavan*, while you make your shoulders dance to the music. Dance to free your rib cage. Your total health will benefit by opening up your rib cage in this movement. It's a partnerships between you and your shoulders, not just an up and down movement. Do it with style. **5 minutes**.

6. Use your open palms to beat your inner thighs. Use the rhythm of *Punjabi Drums* to pace your movement. **3 1/2 minutes**. This self-massage will balance the calcium and magnesium in your body and reduce the effects of old age.

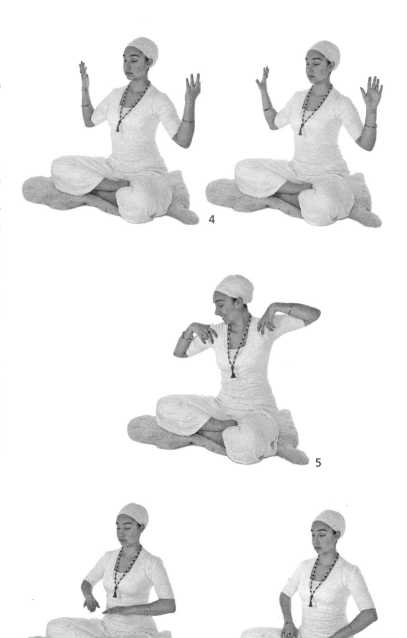

About This Kriya

"To be a woman requires a lot of strength. Your glandular system, your intelligence and your consciousness have to be extraordinarily strong so you can be on the winning side. All the strength of the Universe is within you. It cannot be found outside. Those who do not develop strength from inside cannot get it from outside either." —Yogi Bhajan

WITHSTAND THE PRESSURE OF TIME

JULY 4, 1984

1. Sit in Easy Pose, raise the arms up with bent elbows and begin shaking the whole body. It should be an inward body massage. Every muscle and fiber must shake. Arms, body and head must move. Create your own rhythm and style. Generating heat. **15 minutes**. *This will release toxins from your muscles. Get wild. Shake like an earthquake. It would take hours of massage to get to this point. Cheeks should get red. You must come to the dead end of tiredness.*

2. Come standing up straight. Shake the hips from side to side by bending the knees alternately. Feet can either stay on the ground and hands can dangle loosely, or vigorously twist the hips and jump in the air while pumping your arms. **8 minutes**.
Make this an energetic dance. Your thigh muscles should sweat. This will get rid of toxins, the dirty fat, the tissue deposits. This will get out the old anger in your body.

3. In Easy Pose, extend the arms straight over the head with palms together, arms against the ears. Twist the body left and right. **4 minutes**.
It is a triangular move. If done powerfully, it will release your shoulders.

4. On the hands and knees, lift the left leg straight out behind you. Touch the forehead to the ground and come back up, like push-ups. **52 times**. Repeat with right leg. **52 times**.

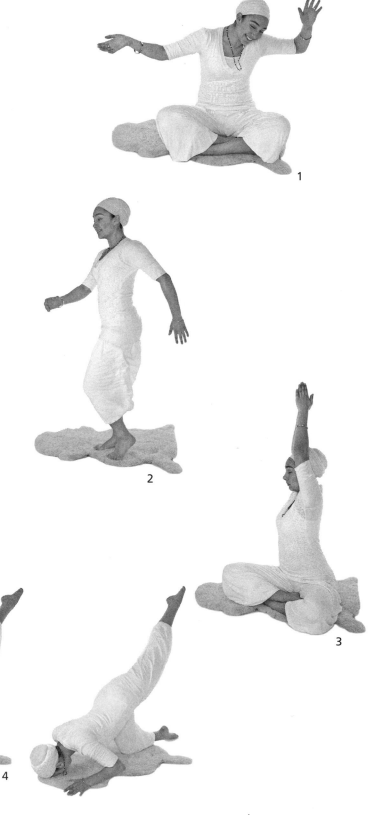

5. Come standing on your knees and bend back into **Camel Pose**, resting the hands on the heels. Then straighten the back up onto the knees. **55 times**.

6. Lie down flat on the back.

    (a) Lift the knees up to the chest and place the hands under the hips. You may elevate the hips with the hands slightly, in order to get the knees to the chest.

    (b) Extend the legs straight out.

    (c) Raise the legs up to 90 degrees. Then bring the knees back to the chest. **108 times**.

This movement gives power for your prana to be controlled by will. It is the movement of the Pavanmuktasana, where the prana is controlled by will.

7. Lie down flat and put both hands over the Heart Center and relax. Sit up and bring the forehead to the knees and relax back down on the back. **26 times**.

8. **Corpse Pose.** Lie down flat on the back for a deep relaxation. If a gong is available, make this a gong meditation. **8 minutes**.
You will become weightless and enjoy it. Relax.

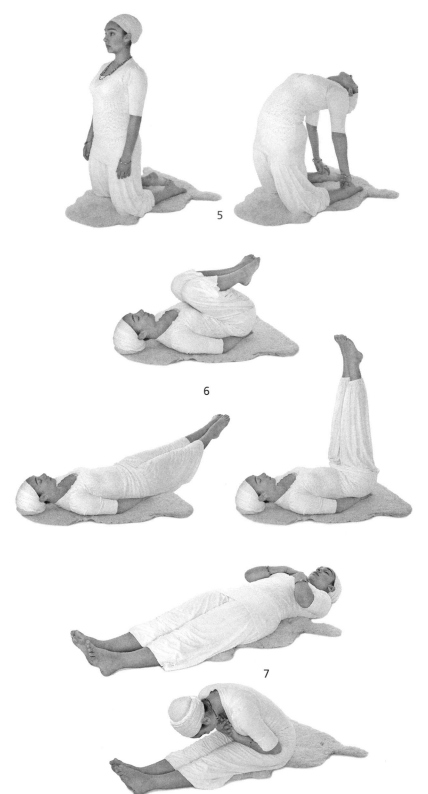

5

6

7

About This Kriya

This is a powerful and energetic kriya for a full tune-up of the nervous system. If the nerves are not tuned-up you will not be able to withstand the pressure of the time. This also works on two problems common to a woman—locked up pelvis and locked shoulders.

MEDITATION FOR **ABSOLUTELY POWERFUL ENERGY**

MAY 17, 1976

POSTURE: Sit in Easy Pose with the spine straight, and a firm Neck Lock.

MUDRA: Interlace the fingers, keeping the Sun (Ring) fingers together pointing upwards. The right thumb is on top. Hold the hands several inches out from the diaphragm, allowing the Sun fingers to be pointing up at 60 degrees.

EYE FOCUS: Eyes are closed.

BREATH & MANTRA: Inhale deeply and powerfully chant the sound:

ONG

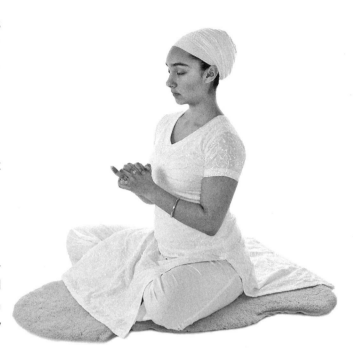

The sound is prolonged and continuous, and created by holding a strong Neck Lock, closing the back of the throat and using the head like a conch. The sound is vibrated through the central subtle nerve channel the *Sushmana*, accessed by vibrating the center of the nose.

When chanting in a group, each person should use her own breath rhythm.

TIME: Unspecified. Suggested practice: 5 or more repetitions.

About This Meditation

The power of this chant, when correctly done, must be experienced to be believed. Only 5 repetitions are necessary to totally elevate the consciousness. When you have a hard day to face, this meditation will give you absolutely powerful energy, and it will balance your most effective computer—the brain. The meditation can also be done when you are able to sleep afterwards. It is the best thing to do for "brain drain."

MEDITATION TO **FIGHT BRAIN FATIGUE** AND LIVE YOUR EXCELLENCE

MARCH 27, 1995

POSTURE & MUDRA: Sit in Easy Pose with the elbows bent and upper arms near the rib cage. The forearms point straight out in front of the body, parallel to the floor. The right palm faces down and the left palm faces up.

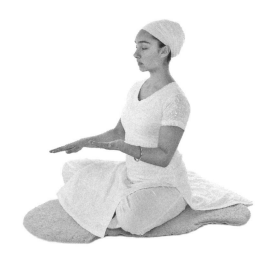

PART ONE

Breathing through the nose, inhale in **8 strokes** and exhale in **8 strokes**. On each stroke of the breath, alternatively move the hands up and down. One hand moves up as the other hand moves down. The movement of the hands is slight, approximately 6-8 inches, as if you are bouncing a ball. Breathe powerfully. Continue for **3 minutes**

Then change the hand position so that the left palm faces downward and the right palm faces upward. Continue for another **3 minutes**.

Then change the hand position again so that the right palm faces down and the left palm faces up. Continue for a final **3 minutes**.

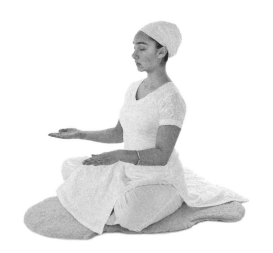

TIME: Total time for this sequence is **9 minutes**. Hold the position and move into Part Two.

PART TWO

Hold the same mudra, and begin long, slow, deep breathing. Close the eyes and focus at the center of the chin. Keep the body perfectly still so it can heal itself. Keep the mind quiet, stilling all thoughts.

TIME: 5 1/2 minutes.

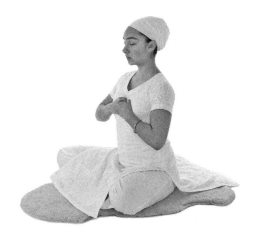

TO END: Inhale deeply, suspend the breath, make the hands into fists and press them strongly against the chest. 15 seconds. Exhale. Inhale deeply, hold the breath, and press the fists against the Navel Point. 15 seconds. Exhale. Inhale deeply, hold the breath, bend the elbows bringing the fists near the shoulders and press the arms firmly against the rib cage, 15 seconds. Exhale and relax.

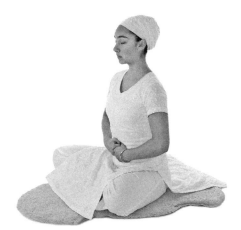

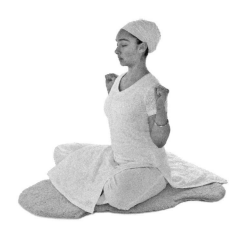

About This Meditation

This exercise balances the diaphragm and fights brain fatigue. It renews the blood supply to the brain and moves the serum in the spine. It also benefits the liver, navel, spleen and lymphatic system.

MEDITATION TO **PREVENT FREAKING OUT**

JUNE 7, 1976

POSTURE: Sit in Easy Pose with a straight spine, and a light Neck Lock.

MUDRA: Interlace the fingers with the right thumb on top. Place the hands at the center of the diaphragm line, touching the body.

EYE FOCUS: Eyes are closed.

BREATH: Concentrate on the breath at the tip of your nose. Notice from which nostril you are breathing. Within **3 minutes** you should know. Then change it. If you are breathing primarily through your left nostril, consciously change to your right nostril. Be sure to keep your shoulders completely relaxed. Practice changing this breath back and forth for as long as you like.

TIME: You may work up to **31 minutes**.

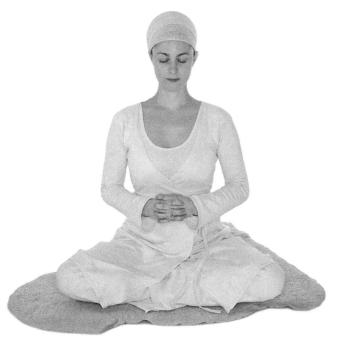

About This Meditation

This meditation will alter your energy by changing your nostril breathing. You can't get out of your body, but you can change its energy. If you are thinking something neurotic and find out that you're breathing through your right nostril, start breathing through your left nostril instead. This will change your energy from *agni* (fire) to *sitali* (cool).

If you are depressed, in a disturbed mental state, start breathing from the right nostril. In 3 minutes you will be a different person. This ability to change nostrils in breathing should be taught to your children within their first 3 years. Exercising this ability can prevent nervous breakdowns.

MEDITATION TO **TRANQUILIZE THE MIND**

FEBRUARY 28, 1979

POSTURE: Sit in Easy Pose with a straight spine, with a light Neck Lock.

MUDRA: With the elbows bent, bring the hands up to meet in front of the body at the level of the heart. The elbows are held up almost to the level of the hands. Bend the Jupiter (index) fingers of each hand in toward the palm, and press them together along the second joint. The Saturn (middle) fingers are extended and meet at the fingertips. The other fingers are curled into the hand. The thumb tips are joined and pointing toward the body. Hold the mudra about 4 inches from the body with the extended fingers pointing away from the body.

EYE FOCUS: Focus on the tip of your nose.

BREATH & MANTRA: Inhale completely and hold the breath while repeating the mantra of your choice **11-21 times**. Exhale, hold the breath out, and repeat the mantra an equal number of times.

TIME: 3 minutes.

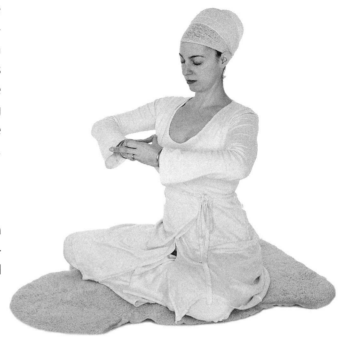

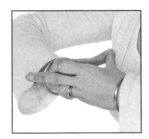

About This Meditation

This meditation will tranquilize the mind within 3 minutes. The hand position is called "the mudra which pleases the mind." Buddha gave it to his disciples for control of the mind.

MEDITATION FOR THE **MOST RESTLESS MIND**
FEBRUARY 19, 1979

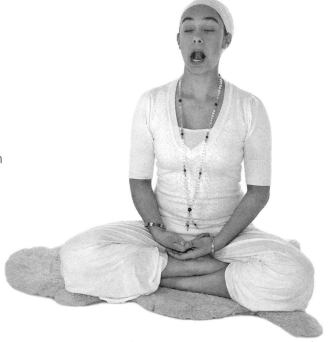

POSTURE: Sit in Easy Pose with a straight spine, with a light Neck Lock.

MUDRA: Relax the arms and hands in any meditative pose.

EYE FOCUS: Focus on the tip of the nose.

BREATH: Open the mouth as wide as possible. Touch the tongue to the upper palate. Breathe through the nose.

TIME: Start with **3 to 5 minutes** of practice, with a maximum of 11 minutes. With practice, it can be done for 31 minutes.

About This Meditation

This meditation gives immediate relief to any wavering, spaced-out mind. When there is so much insanity around that even medical and psychiatric help falls short, this will not. Practicing the kriya gives the capacity to still the most restless mind. Before you recommend it to someone, make sure you've practiced it yourself!

THE TRIPLE MANTRA

The Triple Mantra consists of three mantras which are recited in a monotone, or chanted along with a musical version, in the following sequence:

ONE		
	Aad guray nameh	*I bow to the Primal Guru*
	Jugaad guray nameh	*I bow to the truth throughout the ages*
	Sat guray nameh	*I bow to True Wisdom*
	Siri guroo dayv-ay nameh	*I bow to the great unseen wisdom*

TWO		
	Aad sach	*True in the Primal Beginning*
	Jugaad sach	*True throughout the Ages*
	Haibhee sach	*True even now*
	Naanak hosee bhee sach	*Oh Nanak! Forever and ever True!*

THREE		
	Aad sach	*True in the Primal Beginning*
	Jugaad sach	*True throughout the Ages*
	Haibhai sach	*True even now*
	Naanak hosee bhai sach	*Oh Nanak! Forever and ever True!*

Chant the 'sachhhhh' like the hiss of a snake and feel it in your spine. Part Two is chanted softer than Part Three, which is chanted in a more emphatic tone.

TIME: Chant this mantra for **11, 15, 22,** or **31 minutes** for **40 days** to be able to call upon its power and its promise.

TO END: When you are finished, sit quietly and listen inside. Simply Listen. This is an important part of the meditation.

About This Meditation

The Triple Mantra tunes the mind into the cosmic dance. As this mantra is chanted, the mind talks to itself in a cosmic way. In the process, we connect and surrender to the universal dance of polarities. The Triple mantra reprograms our mind so that we can operate from the Neutral Mind—so that we can move out of duality into the dance of universal polarities. The Triple Mantra clears all types of mental, psychic, and physical obstacles in one's daily life. It protects against accidents. It cuts through opposing vibrations, thoughts, words and actions. It strengthens your mind and magnetic field and keeps negativity away. This mantra opens us up to be guided by faith instead of fear. If we are guided by fear, we block ourselves. If we are guided by faith, we open ourselves up to expansion and creation.

The mantra used in Part One puts you into the mode of acceptance and surrender to Universal Truth and wisdom. It surrounds you with a powerful light of protection. Your aura protects you by becoming light and clear.

Parts Two and Three are forms of the same mantra. They align our energy with the truth. Together they achieve a balance between passive and active. The complete mantra solidifies the cosmic dance within us. The form used in Part 2, the *Bhee* puts us into an accepting, allowing and surrender mode. This is the last four lines of the *Mul Mantra*. This mantra embodies the vibration of stability and eternal truth, that which never changes. The form used in Part 3, the *Bhai* is active. This mantra embodies the active, creative, evolutionary aspect of the universe. It breaks through energetic blocks and opens the space for things to happen. It also aligns your energy field so you can attract opportunities and take advantage of them.

THE "LAST RESORT" MEDITATION

JUNE 15, 1982

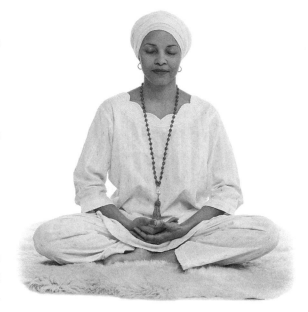

POSTURE: Sit in Easy Pose with spine straight. Have the hands in the lap, palms up, right hand resting in left, thumb tips touching.

EYE FOCUS: Eyes are closed.

MANTRA: Chant the *Wahe Guru Wahe Jio* mantra 8 times on one breath. Chant in a monotone:

> *WHAA-HAY GUROO   WHAA-HAY GUROO*
> *WHAA-HAY GUROO WHAA-HAY JEE-O*

Breathe very deeply in order to complete the cycle, which will take approximately 45 seconds. Release the breath very slowly as you chant. If at first the breath doesn't hold for the full 8 repetitions, stop, breathe, and begin again. Build up your capacity.

TIME: Start with **11 minutes** maximum. Gradually increase to 22 minutes, then 33 minutes.

About This Meditation

"This meditation brings relaxation, strength, and mental clarity. It brings soul talk—the infinite capacity to experience the power of your soul right on the spot. It enables you to keep giving to a friend. If you do this meditation for 11 minutes a day for six months, you will experience the cosmos. You can talk to God. If you do it for a year, God will come and listen to you!

Remember: you breathe, you live, because there is a soul in you. The soul is a tiny tender light in your body. I'm giving you a meditation today. I call it the "Last Meditation." It is not that it is the last meditation I will teach you. But understand it's essence. It is for when life doesn't work for you, and you don't want to go to anybody and say, 'I'm going crazy, please help me.' I understand that sometimes personal image is very important. Despite how depressed you may be, just do this meditation and find out for yourself: Kundalini Yoga is a science and an art which can totally make a human being healthy, happy, and holy.

The mantra means: "You are beloved of my Soul, Oh God." It causes a very subtle rub against the center of the palate, and stimulates the 32nd meridian, known in the West as the Christ Meridian, and in the East as Sattvica Buddha Bindh. The tongue and lips correspond to the Sun and Moon in their movement. The practice of this kriya will enable you to think right, act right, see right, look at yourself, imagine and meditate. Everything else follows. You will wipe out a lot of negativity.

Many things will happen in my absence which you need to survive through. Even if you are the dumbest of the dummies and nobody wants to buy you for 20 cents, if you can do this meditation correctly, you will come out with the best of yourself. Please participate with heart and mind, and see that you do it."

— Yogi Bhajan

Part Three

THE SACRED FEMININE
& THE DIVINE MOTHER

Creative Consciousness & the Longing to Merge

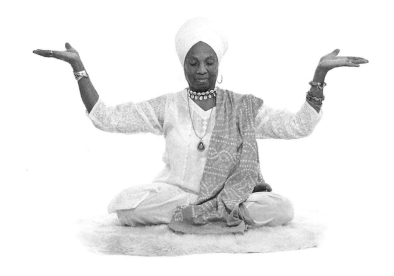

SEXUALITY & CREATIVITY

IGNITING THE SPARK

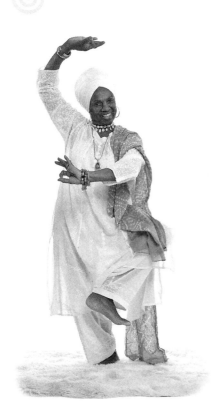

WOMAN RECEIVES, CONCEIVES and creates—that is her basic nature. Whether conceiving through the passion of a man's seed and creating a child, or creating whole and healthy environments, or cultivating her own grace and perpetuating it—woman is the embodiment of the creativity of humankind.

I USED TO TELL MY TWO BEAUTIFUL DAUGHTERS that if God had given me the power to change the world, to heal one thing on this planet and in the psyche of humanity, which would make the most difference, it would be this: a woman's sexuality, creativity, and power would be recognized and integrated with her grace, her purity, and her creativity; and no longer seen as something to be simply "penetrated," entitled to, or exploited.

Woman receives, conceives and creates—that is her basic nature. Whether conceiving through the passion of a man's seed and creating a child, or creating whole and healthy environments, or cultivating her own grace and perpetuating it—woman is the embodiment of the creativity of humankind. She is the universal creativity, the Universal Womb.

The dynamic, ever-present, creative consciousness of a woman manifests the longing to merge—the urge to merge—one of the most powerful forces of the human psyche. What will she do with this awesome power? If her consciousness is clear, connected and listening to the voice of her soul, this longing will attract that which will serve her life and her grace—and never destroy it. This is a primal force within the woman and a dynamic reality in her life. In fact, the source of this attraction is her core self-identity: the recognition of herself as the embodiment of the Sacred Feminine, in all of her many dimensions.

There is no need for duality between her passion and her purity. Instead, her passion can serve her purity. Jiwan Joti Kaur Khalsa, PhD, in her book *The Art of Making Sex Sacred* says:

"Now is a time exploding with spirituality. In the Piscean Age, due to religious dogma, we lost our connection to our soul, our Divine Self, and our sacredness. In the Aquarian Age, we are reconnecting to our soul through spiritual experiences. What we are truly seeking is intimacy, meaningful connection, and fulfillment. We see this searching in all aspects of our current culture. Yoga is a household word. Prayer is an accepted method for healing. Man, nature and Higher Force are regarded as One, deserving equal respect, consideration and protection. Those seeking spirituality are quickly viewing the lustful sex sold to us in movies and books as shallow, limited, and sometimes abusive. Doesn't it make complete sense that we want our sexual experience to reflect our expanding consciousness? The concept of sacred sex represents the reclaiming of our role as divine beings merging through intimate communion with God and another person."

Conceiving a Passionate & Pure Life

To conceive a passionate life filled with grace, vitality, and happiness for herself and those around her, woman needs to be relaxed, secure, and in command of her domain. By the way, a wise man will protect these qualities—and receive the benefits!

A woman has three creative capacities that work in unison: the power of Bij Gupha, the power of Gyan Gupha, and the power of her Arcline. ("*Gupha*" means "cave.")

The Bij Gupha is the "seed cave." In this *gupha* is her power of receiving a man and conceiving his seed through sexual intercourse, with all of its delights and responsibilities. In this "seed cave" the play of masculine and feminine find their merger and ecstasy. In this realm, a woman needs vitality, stamina, vibrant health, confidence, and heart, as well as a balanced chakra system.

The Gyan Gupha is the "cave of knowledge and wisdom." In this *gupha* is the power of the Word—her mouth, her tongue, and her subtle creativity. It is here, through mantra and japa, that she churns the power of her Word. The power of her own masculine and feminine aspects merge to create ecstasy and integrity in the reality and creativity of her Word.

Finally, we come to her Aura, and particularly the nucleus of her Aura—the Arcline. The Arcline is her protection and projection, beaming powerfully from her essence, commanding her own domain, projecting her desires, both conscious and unconscious, and serving to protect her as an energetic filter. A woman has two Arclines: One is shared by both men and women, the one from ear to ear, like a halo. But a woman's second Arcline, from nipple to nipple, gives her an enhanced capacity for sensitivity, attraction, and subtle intuition. And news flash, dear ones: as you receive and conceive a man into your aura, especially, but not only, through sexual intercourse, your Arcline is deeply imprinted with his essence. As Yogi Bhajan says: "A woman should understand her own security before she indulges in relationships with men, because all relationships are very deeply imprinted in her."

A woman's Arcline is her best friend. Serve and care for your Arcline through sadhana and meditation. Ask yourself, "Have you cleared and strengthened your Arcline today?"

THE KRIYAS AND MEDITATIONS gathered for this section are both subtle and commanding. The **Sex Energy Transformation series** and the **Complete Workout for the Elementary Being: Har Aerobic Kriya** get down to healing, balancing, and invoking the basic power of your sexual, creative energy. Did you know that according to yogic tradition, the main use of the sexual energy was to repair and rejuvenate the organs of the body? If the body is well cared for and nutrition is well-balanced, one maintains potency and sexual interest throughout one's lifespan. It's all about the *ojas*. Check it out.

The **Meditation for the Arcline: Realize Your Power** is one of the most intuitive meditations I have ever experienced. In these few minutes, you as a woman realize how you make things move, including this "neutral form" called a man. It is subtle, and cultivates patience through the power of the rhythm of your subtle projection, creating, commanding, quietly but confidently, slowly but surely, over time.

Becoming Crystal Clear adjusts the proper flow between the Third and Fourth Chakras, so that you can live through the heart, strong and clear. Life is about crystallization, not sublimation. Crystallize your Self and shine brightly—live creatively!

Meditation for the Fifth Chakra heals your Throat Chakra so that your Gyan Gupha can function optimally. The hormonal balance that results from a balanced thyroid delivers a sense of well-being, and a clear and bright face and grace.

With the **Adi Shakti Meditation for Vitality** you consolidate, embody, and project the power of the Adi Shakti as your own identity, your own power. No nonsense penetrates this field.

Allow your true grace and power, your unique qualities as a woman, to inform your creativity and vitality. Become a purposeful and self-contained woman, integrated in her sexuality and living in her majesty.

GURU RAJ KAUR KHALSA
VANCOUVER, B.C. CANADA

SEX ENERGY TRANSFORMATION

OCTOBER 3, 1979

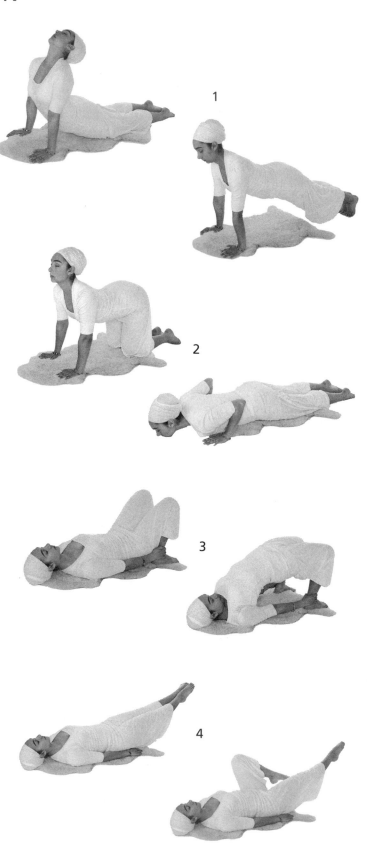

1. **Cobra Pose & Front Platform Pose**. Lying on the stomach, place hands under the shoulders with palms flat. Stretch up into Cobra by elongating the spine, lifting the chest and heart up, dropping the shoulders, and stretching the head back. Straighten the arms. Inhale and raise the hips straight off the ground into Front Platform. Exhale, lower the hips back down into Cobra. Repeat **26 times**. Relax on the stomach for **2 minutes**.
Chant ONG on the inhale and SOHUNG on the exhale. This will keep a rhythm and help keep the mind focused. ONG means "the Infinite, creative consciousness." SOHUNG means "I am Thou".

2. **Cow Pose**. On the hands and knees, with hands shoulder-width apart, fingers facing forward, knees directly under the hips, tilt the pelvis, arching the spine down, head and neck stretched back. Stretch forward on the exhale, allowing the hips and the chin to touch the ground. Keep the head up and the arms bent. Inhale back into Cow Pose. Repeat **26 times**.
Continue to Chant ONG — on the forward motion; and SOHUNG — when back in Cow Pose.
Move immediately into the next exercise.

3. **Pelvic Lifts**. Immediately without resting, lie down on the back. Bend the knees and grasp the ankles. The soles of the feet stay on the ground next to the hips. Inhale—lift the hips. Exhale—relax down. Repeat **26 times**. Rest for **2 minutes**. Repeat **26 more times**.

4. Immediately extend both legs and raise them 18 inches from the floor. Begin Long Deep Breathing for **30 seconds**. Breathe powerfully. Begin a piston motion with the legs; bring one knee to the chest, then the other with each deep inhale. Continue alternating with this push-pull action for up to **1 minute**. Inhale— extend both legs straight out for **5 seconds**. Relax.

5. Lie on the back. Bring the soles of the feet together and grab them with the hands. Rock forward and back on the spine for **30–45 seconds**.

6. **Deep relaxation** for **2 minutes**.

7. **Stretch Pose**. Lie on the back with the feet together, toes pointed. Flatten the lower back. Place hands palms down over the thighs, pointing towards the toes. Lift the head up, apply Neck Lock and look at the toes. Lift the feet up 6 inches and balance in this position and for up to **7 minutes**. Inhale deeply, exhale, hold the breath out and apply *mulbandh*. Hold the breath out as long as possible. Repeat the inhale, exhale, *mulbandh* **4 more times**. Relax down.

8. **Deep Relaxation**. Completely relax for **5 minutes** letting the energy circulate. Think of God and God-consciousness. Feel unlimited. After 5 minutes come back from relaxation by chanting *"God and Me, Me and God, are One"* about **12 times**, raising the pitch and volume gradually across these repetitions. Inhale deeply, hold for **15 seconds**, then exhale. Start the chant again but very powerfully. Chant loudly from the Navel Point and solar plexus. Keep the eyes closed. Do not feel shy.

TO END: Inhale and exhale **8 times**. Then inhale, suspend the breath and raise the legs to 90 degrees. Hold for **15 seconds**. Exhale and relax.

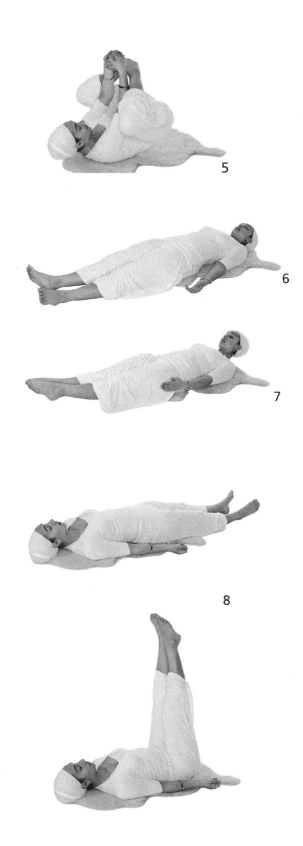

9. **Pranayam Sequence**. Sit in Easy Pose. Use the thumb and little finger of one hand to close alternate nostrils. There should be no break between this sequence of *pranayam*—each flows into the next.

(a) Inhale through the left nostril, exhale through the right. Meditate at the base of the spine and pull *mulbandh*. On the inhale, mentally vibrate *Sat*; on the exhale vibrate *Naam*. Continue for **1 minute**.

(b) Breath of Fire, inhaling through the left nostril, exhaling through the right for **1 minute**.

(c) Inhale and exhale through the left nostril only, moderately fast for about **15 seconds**.

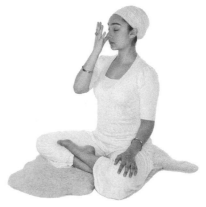

9

(d) Begin Breath of Fire through the left nostril for **15 seconds**, then through the right nostril for **15 seconds**. Then again through the left nostril for **5 seconds** and through the right for **5 seconds**.

TO END: Release the hand and inhale through both nostrils and hold **5 seconds**. Exhale, holding the breath out for **30 seconds**. As you suspend the breath out, flow smoothly through this visualization: mentally repeat the mantra *SAT NAAM*, visualize the sound following an upward spiral along the spine. Then visualize *SAT* going down both sides of the spine, entering the base of the spine and *NAAM* rising up the middle of the spine. Close the mind to every other thing and concentrate. Now is the time. One or two more times, inhale deeply and exhale then repeat the mental visualization.

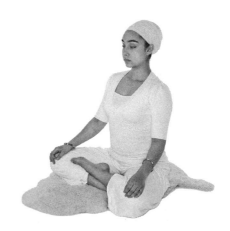

10. Chant this mantra in the following manner:

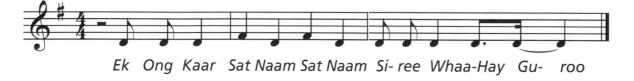

Ek Ong Kaar Sat Naam Sat Naam Si- ree Whaa-Hay Gu- roo

When chanting *SAT NAM* and *GURU*, apply and release *mulbandh*. Gradually the *mulbandh* will become so strong and locked that it will be easy to hold throughout the entire chant. Continue chanting for **6 minutes**.

TO END: Inhale—hold for **15 seconds**. Exhale and relax.

About This Kriya

In our culture, we are taught to view sex in terms of pleasure and reproduction. We are not taught how important moderation in sex is in order to maintain our health and nerve balance. Sexual experience in the correct consciousness can give you the experience of God and bliss, but before that can ever occur you must charge your sexual batteries and nurture real potency. The seminal fluids produced in the male and the fluids produced in the female contain high concentrations of minerals and elements that are crucial to proper nerve balance and brain functioning. According to yogic tradition, these sexual fluids called *ojas*, are reabsorbed by the body, if allowed to mature, and the minerals and nutrient elements taken into the spinal fluid. Running your brain without the *ojas* is like running a car without oil—you wear out quickly. It was said that the main use of the sexual energy was to repair and rejuvenate the organs of the body. If the body is well cared for and nutrition is well-balanced, the yogi maintains potency and sexual interest throughout one's lifespan.

It is common to see potency waning as early as in the 40s. This kriya will generate sexual energy and transmute it into *ojas* for healing and continued sexual vitality. The first three exercises activate the Second Chakra; then the Navel Point and lower spine. Exercise 3 is especially effective for relieving tension and problems of the ovaries. Exercises 4 and 5 move the energy out of the digestive system. Exercise 7 distributes the energy from the Navel Point above the solar plexus to the Heart Center. Exercise 9 uses *pranayam* to completely open your psychic channels and move the kundalini energy all the way to the highest chakras. Exercise 10 uses the kundalini energy in the mantra to project the mind into the infinity of the Cosmos and beyond our normal earthly consciousness.

COMPLETE WORKOUT FOR THE **ELEMENTARY BEING** HAR AEROBIC KRIYA

1. Standing with feet comfortably apart, clap the hands over the head **8 times**. Each time you clap, chant *HAR* with the tip of the tongue.

2. Bend over from the hips. Slap the ground hard with the hands **8 times**. With each pat, chant *HAR* with the tip of the tongue.

3. Stand up straight up with arms out to the sides parallel to the ground. Raise and lower the arms, patting the air, one foot up and one foot below the shoulder height, as you chant *HAR* with the tip of the tongue. **8 times**.

4. Still standing, jump and crisscross the arms and legs chanting *HAR*, both as the arms and legs cross, and when they are out at the sides, for a total of **8 chants** of *HAR*.

5. Come into **Archer Pose** with the right leg forward, left leg back. Bend the right knee, extending in and out of the full stretch of the position, chanting *HAR* each time you bend forward. **8 times**. Switch sides, with the left leg extended forward, chanting *HAR* each time you bend forward. **8 times**.

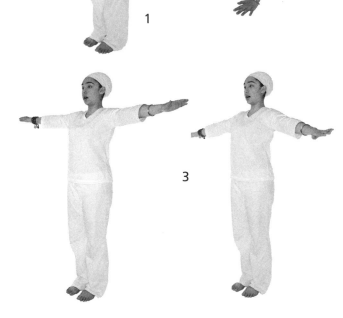

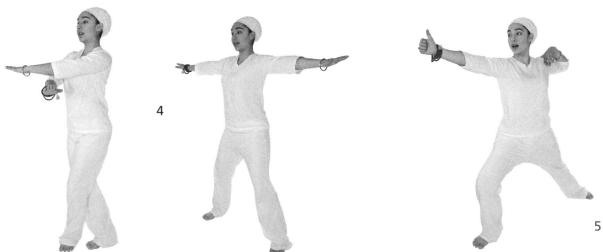

6. Repeat crisscross jumping as in Exercise 4.

7. Stretch the arms over the head. Arch the back as you bend backwards, chanting *HAR* each time you bend back. **8 times**.

8. Repeat crisscross jumping as in Exercise 4.

9. With the arms straight up over the head, bend to the left **4 times** and bend to the right **4 times**, chanting *HAR* each time you bend. Keep the arms close to the head.

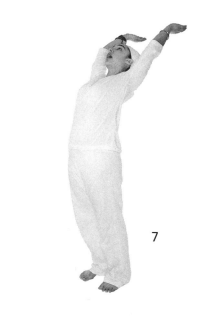

7

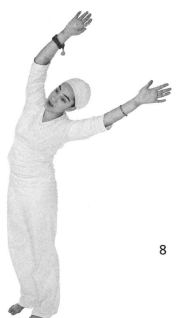

8

About This Kriya

This set is to be done very quickly, moving from exercise to exercise with no break. When done properly it is a great aerobic workout. Repeat the sequence **5 times**.

MEDITATION FOR THE **ARCLINE: REALIZE YOUR POWER**

JULY 3, 1996

POSTURE: Sit in Easy Pose with a straight spine.

MUSIC: *Rhythms of Gatka* recording by Matamandir Singh.

PART ONE

MUDRA: Make fists. Extend the Jupiter and Saturn (Index and middle) fingers straight, fingertips touching. Hold the Sun and Mercury (ring and pinkie) fingers down with the thumb. Bend the elbows and place them into the sides of the body.

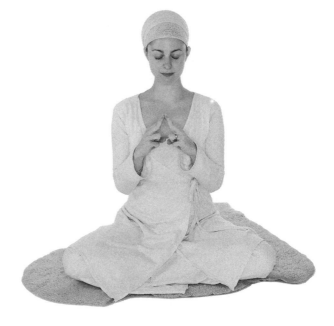

EYE FOCUS: Focus at the tip of the nose.

MOVEMENT:

(a) Bring the two hands with palms facing each other in front of the chest, touching only the extended fingertips of the right hand with the extended fingertips of the left hand.

(b) Swing the hands out to the sides, palms facing forward, with a space of about 24 inches between the hands. The extended fingers of the right and left hands will be at 45-degree angles. With each major beat of the drum, touch the fingers together in front of the chest.

Swing the arms from (a) to (b) in a sweeping, continuous motion. There are no breaks in the movement.

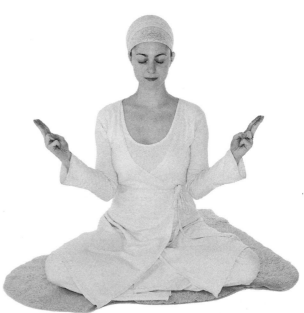

MANTRA: Chant *HAR* from the Navel Point as the fingers touch.

TIME: Done in class for **14 minutes**.

PART TWO

MUDRA & MOVEMENT: Make fists. Extend the Jupiter (index) and Saturn (middle) fingers straight, and together. Hold the Sun and Mercury (ring and pinkie) fingers down with the thumb. Raise the right arm straight up in the air, with no bend in the elbow. Palm faces forward, and the two extended fingers point straight up. Your right arm will be hugging the right ear. Place the left hand across the Heart Center, palm facing down, lower arm parallel to the ground.

MENTAL FOCUS: Start moving the hands mentally (as in Part One), without actually moving the hands. Make the body into a solid state. Make absolutely no movement, move no muscle. Just move mentally.

EYE FOCUS: The eyes are closed.

MUSIC: *Rhythms of Gatka* recording by Matamandir Singh.

TIME: Done in class for about **2 minutes**.

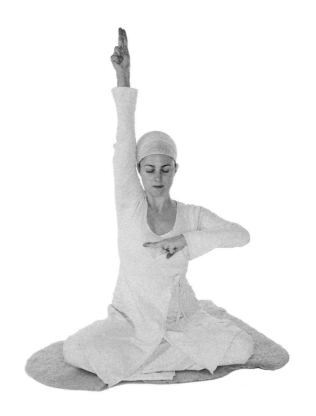

About This Meditation

All people have an Arcline as part of the aura, which extends from ear to ear over the brow—like a halo. These Arclines serve as a center of protection and projection for the individual. Women have two Arclines, the one from ear to ear, and the second from nipple to nipple across the Heart Center. The Heart Center Arcline in imprinted with the experiences a woman has gone through in her life.

This meditation can help you to realize the power you have as a woman. If you can make your body physically standardized and have the mental power to cover the standard of it, you can move anything. What is it that moves? Mind over body. It's a simple development. It's something you should not forget.

If a female doesn't know how the mind can conquer and work on a body, she shall never be in a position to work on her own children. You must know how to move an object, and you must know how to convey the subject; and you must know how to move the object and how to convey the subject of the mammal called male. These are the faculties and facilities given a female by God. To do that, you need to understand *Purusha* in a neutral form. Men are not what you think they are. Men are not what their mothers thought they are, men are not what the environments think they are. Man is a neutral identity. Whatever you as a woman reflect, that shall be.

BECOMING CRYSTAL CLEAR

OCTOBER 2, 1985

1. Bring the arms straight out to the sides, parallel to the ground, with the palms facing forward. Begin alternately bringing the palms in as if to beat the chest, but do not touch the chest. Breath of Fire will automatically develop from the motion, if you do it correctly and powerfully. Imagine that you are pulling pranic energy in with each motion of the hands. **6 1/2 minutes**.

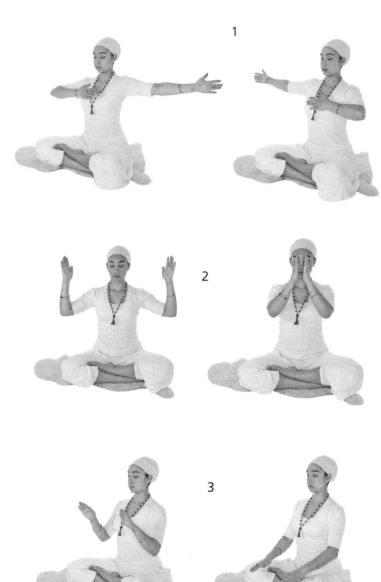

2. Bring the hands in forcefully as if to clap them in front of the face, but do not touch the hands together. Combine force and control in your movement. **2 1/2 minutes**.

3. Move both hands up and down at the same time as if bouncing a ball with each hand, and imagine that you are bouncing energy against the ground. Breath of Fire. **30 seconds**.

4. Lie down flat and put both hands against the Navel Point. Press hard. Raise the heels up 6 inches and hold. Think you are divine or feel sexy, but keep the heels six inches off the ground. **6 1/2 minutes**.

5. Lie down and go to sleep. Imagine that your body is filled with light. Focus at your Navel Point. Listen to the recording of *Dhan Dhan Ram Das Gur* called *Naad, the Blessing* by Sangeet Kaur. After **8 minutes** begin to sing along using the power of the navel for another **7 minutes**.

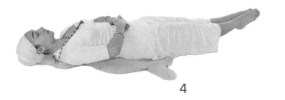

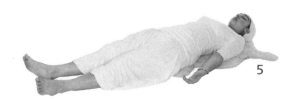

MEDITATION FOR THE **FIFTH CHAKRA**

FEBRUARY 19, 1991

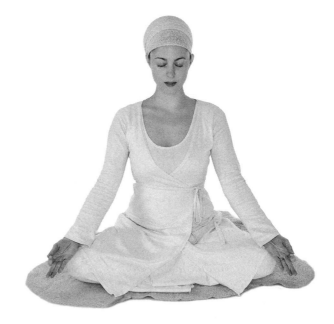

POSTURE: Sit in Easy Pose with a straight spine, and a firm Neck Lock.

MUDRA: The arms are straight and the hands are in Gyan Mudra. The wrists are resting on the knees, palms up.

EYE FOCUS: Focus at the tip of the nose.

MANTRA: Chant the *Humee Hum* mantra with the root of the tongue, and holding the firm Neck Lock.

HUMEE HUM BRAHM HUM

MUSIC: Nirinjan Kaur's recording of *Humee Hum Brahm Hum* can be used or chant in monotone.

TIME: 22 minutes.

About This Meditation

Do it 11 minutes daily for 18 months and your face will not age. It will give endurance, intuition and reverse disease.

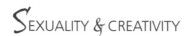
ADI SHAKTI MEDITATION FOR VITALITY

JULY 10, 1998

PART ONE

POSTURE: Sit in Easy Pose with a straight spine.

MUDRA: Bend the elbows down by the sides. Bring the hands into Ravi Mudra, Sun (ring) finger held down with the thumb, the palms face forward and the fingers point straight up. Keep the other fingers straight.
Important: The wrists are at the level of the shoulders, with the hands in line with the ears. Make sure the spine is kept very straight, and Neck Lock engaged.

EYES: Eyes are closed.

MANTRA: Chant along with the Kundalini Bhakti Mantra (Adi Shakti, Namo, Namo.) The recording by Gurudass Kaur is played. *(See page 18 for this mantra.)*

TIME: 31 minutes.

TO END: Inhale, keep the posture steady, and move immediately into Part Two.

PART TWO

MUDRA & MANTRA: Keep the same mudra, don't move at all—begin chanting *HAR* aloud, pulling in on the Navel Point with each recitation. The recording *Tantric Har* is used.

TIME: 4 minutes.

TO END: Inhale very deeply. Hold **15-20 seconds**. Exhale through the mouth in a whistle. Inhale a second time, very deeply, hold **15-20 seconds**. Whistle out every bit of breath you can. Inhale a third time, and squeeze your entire being. Hold and squeeze **10-15 seconds**. Cannon fire out through the mouth. Relax.

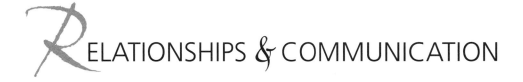

RELATIONSHIPS & COMMUNICATION

REDEFINING INTERCOURSE

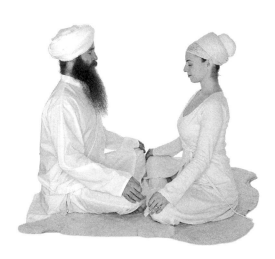

COMMUNICATION AS AN INTERCOURSE can be described as the play of Bhakti and Shakti. Devotional listening and empowered communication can manifest a most rare thing —true merger between two souls.

"IN THE BEGINNING WAS THE WORD"—and from that word all things are created, even today. Communication in relationships is such a vital skill for every woman to master; it encompasses not only the spoken word, but the silent gesture, the look that can zero out any man. Yogi Bhajan spoke about communication as the ultimate intercourse. Communication with God, with your Self and your soul, and with your partner—the beautiful dance of intimacy, penetration, and merger—is true intercourse, a way to achieve celestial bliss and oneness with the Universe. Communication as an intercourse can be described as the play of Bhakti and Shakti. Devotional listening and empowered communication can manifest a most rare thing—true merger between two souls.

The first principle of communication is honesty within yourself. If you are afraid to look and listen to the hidden parts of your own personality, you'll never be able to be vulnerable and open to another person or allow them to really see you—and to be seen is to be loved. So we open this chapter with a meditation on the **Naad and How to Communicate Your Honest Self**. Another key component to healthy communication is listening; so we have included the **Meditation to Experience the Naad**, which builds the practice of listening. The art of truly listening, that is, listening without your own agenda, listening without planning what you're going to say next, listening with an open heart is so beautiful, especially in a marriage; but it can also be applied in any situation where creative communication is necessary to successfully negotiate win-win terms. Speaking honestly and directly, and listening intuitively and deeply, will open the door to deeper intimacy and true intercourse in your relationships.

We have included a few meditations for partners, to help break through communication blocks and build relationship. Practicing together generates a powerful intimacy and cultivates a deepening bond even as it builds up each person, individually. We close the chapter with the *shabd* practice, **Sopurkh**, which uplifts your own relationship to the divine and builds that identity within your partner.

Apply these meditations to your practice and to your life. Master the art of true intercourse and merge with your Self, with your partner, and with God. This is the juice of life! This is the art of living! This is the ultimate practice—*grist yog*—in which the ego is slowly ground down, the personality is refined and the two become one.

SAT PURKH KAUR KHALSA
ESPAÑOLA, NEW MEXICO

NAAD MEDITATION TO **COMMUNICATE YOUR HONEST SELF**

SEPTEMBER 1983

PART ONE

POSTURE: Sit in an Easy Pose, with a light Neck Lock.

EYES: The eyes are closed, focus at the Brow Point.

MUDRA: Bend the arms and raise the hands next to the shoulders. The wrists are straight and the palms face forward. Begin to alternately press the thumb tip to the index finger tip and then to the ring finger tip. Press with about 5 pounds of pressure.

MANTRA: As you rhythmically alternate the fingers, chant the sounds:

> *SAA* – pressing the index finger
> *RAY* – pressing the ring finger

The sound of the chant is a steady, brisk monotone, emphasizing the movement of the tongue and mouth. Feel the pulse of the sound and the energy changing in the body. Continue in a steady pace.

TIME: 31 minutes.

TO END: Inhale and hold as long as it is comfortable. Exhale through the mouth and keep it out with the mouth open. Inhale through the nose again. Hold the breath in for 30 seconds, exhale through the mouth and keep it open for 20 seconds. Inhale deeply and hold the breath for 30 seconds and relax as you exhale through the mouth.

PART TWO

(a) Select a partner and discuss honestly the topic: *"Why don't you believe me?"* Discuss this for **3-15 minutes**.
(b) Assess yourself: *"Am I satisfied or disappointed in this communication?"*
(c) Use the right hand with the palm open to slap the hand of your partner. You both try to slap the hands. As you do this, look at each other's eyes and speak obnoxiously for **3 minutes**.
(d) Immediately put a giant smile on your face. Keep the smile there. Shake the hand of your partner in a simple friendly rhythm for **3 minutes**. Then thank your partner and relax.

About This Meditation

Good communication expresses the real you. It projects the whole self. It discharges your honest self. Clear communication is fearless and does not need anything from the person to whom you are speaking. When you speak out of neediness you distort the real message of your heart. This meditation lets you know where your heart is and what is in it.

This meditation changes the chemistry of the brain. All communication is based on the chemistry and interchange within the brain. The fingertips are points of stimulation for the different areas of the brain. The *naad* rhythm opens creativity and sensitivity to speak from the heart.

MEDITATION FOR CONSCIOUS COMMUNICATION

FEBRUARY 4, 1992

POSTURE: Sit straight in Easy Pose.

PART ONE

EYES: Eyes look down, focusing clearly on each word without having to move the paper, creating a light Neck lock. Peripheral vision will catch the outline of the nose. Fix the optical nerve to make the pituitary become focused and directive, not negative or reactive. This is the first principle for success in this meditation. Fix the eyes.

MANTRA: *Say Saraswati.* Hold the mantra sheet in your right hand. These are Yogi Bhajan's words put to music by Nirinjan Kaur Khalsa under his supervision.

MUDRA: Hold the paper in front of you, as if you are holding a sheet of music. Do not lean in your posture or move. Sit comfortably, and pick the angle of your arm that lets you detect the outline of the nose as you focus clearly on each word you recite.

TIME: 23 minutes.

PART TWO

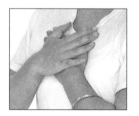

MUDRA: Press the hands on the Heart Center, left palm on the heart, right palm resting on the left hand, eyes tightly closed. Chant for **8 minutes**.

TO END: Inhale deeply. Hold the breath for 20 seconds, pull in the navel and concentrate. Exhale. Repeat for 20 seconds, then 30 seconds.

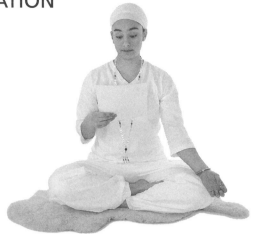

Say Saraswatee Sar-rang
Hay Bhagvatee Har-rang
La Lakhshmee Nar-ring
Karn Kar-an Kar-ring
Dayv Maa-haa Dayv Dayv-uh
Sarab Shaktee Seva
Tarn Taran Tar-ring
Neel Narayan Nar-ring
Guroo Dayv Dayv-ing
Sarab Lok Sev-ing

Goddess of Love — Happiness
Shakti Power — Victory
Goddess of Wealth — Prosperity
God's Three Aspects — Fulfillment
Nurtures the Experience of Totality
The God of Gods, the Infinite One
Under and Over, God Is Love
All Creation, Serving

About This Meditation

This special meditation uses the *Say Saraswati* mantra to invoke the power of the *naad* to lock the brain and mind into a new pattern. The posture used demonstrates a style and technique of meditation that is very technically effective. This shines light on many ancient practices where people would read sacred texts in a manner that assured deep transformation. When we meditate, we look at the tip of the nose because it captures the function of the pituitary so that its responses do not simply react to each wandering thought and feeling. If the pituitary is off, not locked in with you, then two thirds of the time your mind will wander. We don't want the mind to move. We want it to be in control. The moment the optical nerve is locked on anything within the sight of the nose, you are in control.

These affirmations are Yogi Bhajan's: *"Their permutation and combination is according to meridian points in the upper palate which stimulates the hypothalamus. The hypothalamus will react and act with the glandular system and move the pituitary from the inside naturally, not from the outside. Therefore there is no breathing involved with it. The moment the pituitary is forced to take a certain movement of its own secretion, it will affect the glandular system. It will change the radiation cycle of the pineal, the little medical stone in the brain. This is the science of the naad, and you will experience it."*

Both the English and Sanskrit sounds used in this mantra are true to the *naad*. If you simply do it the result will be definite. You will find the next day that your way of speaking has changed.

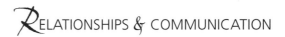

VENUS KRIYAS

How to Practice Venus Kriyas

Venus Kriyas are Kundalini Yoga exercises done with a partner, usually a partner of the opposite sex. Although Venus Kriyas are less intense than White Tantric Yoga, they fall into the category of a more advanced Kundalini Yoga practice, because they intensify the experience of the exercise through the polarities of the male-female interaction. So, adhere to the following guidelines when teaching or practicing Venus Kriyas:

- Always tune in with the Adi Mantra: *Ong Namo Guru Dev Namo* before practicing Venus Kriyas.
- Venus Kriyas are not done to sensually or sexually seduce one's partner. They are done from a state of elevation, to elevate the relationship and the polarities to a purity and their highest vibration. If done with the wrong intention, they lose their effectiveness and in fact, it can be more damaging than helpful.
- Limit the exercise to 3 minutes (unless specifically taught otherwise by Yogi Bhajan.)

Teaching Venus Kriyas

If you are a Kundalini Yoga teacher, and are going to teach Venus Kriyas follow these guidelines:

- It is best to reserve Venus Kriyas only for those with Kundalini Yoga experience. Use your judgement to assess when your students have the disicpline to practice Venus Kriyas. In Venus Kriyas, the energetic and sensory connections of the partners are used to elevate the sexual and sensory energy to a connection based on awareness and the capacity to see the sacred in the other.
- Do not line up in lines as in Tantric Yoga. Two people can sit together anywhere. If you line up, then the energy is shared diagonally. That is not the intention of Venus Kriyas. The energy is only intended to be shared between partners.
- Do not create an entire class using Venus Kriyas. Just use one or two along with a Kundalini Yoga kriya. Yogi Bhajan often added a short Venus Kriya to his Friday classes, to honor the ruling planet Venus.

VENUS KRIYA TO **GET RID OF GRUDGES**

POSTURE: Sit back to back with your partner. Adjust your backs so that they are touching each other, from the bottom to the top of the spine.

MUDRA: Bend the knees and pull the legs to the chest with your arms.

FOCUS: Meditate on your heart. Concentrate on the beating of your heart. Hear it. Meditate on the Sun. Bring this warmth into your heart. Burn out all the bitterness you have felt throughout all the years.

TIME: Continue for **3 minutes**.

TO END: Inhale, exhale, and relax.

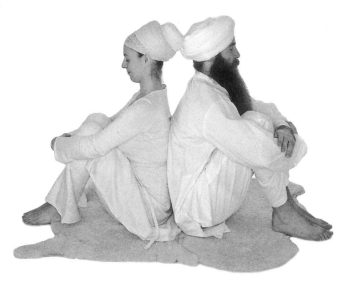

CLEAR THE CLOUDS & ELIMINATE FEAR

POSTURE: Sit back to back in Easy Pose. Adjust your backs so that they are touching each other, from the bottom to the top of the spine.

MANTRA & MUDRA: Chant the Panj Shabd:

SAA TAA NAA MAA

As you chant *SAA*, touch the index finger to the thumb. On *TAA*, touch the middle finger to the thumb. On *NAA*, touch the ring finger to the thumb. On *MAA*, touch the pinkie finger to the thumb. As you chant each syllable, visualize energy entering the top of the head and then moving in an "L" shaped course from the top of your head out through your Third Eye, projecting out into Infinity. *(See Kirtan Kriya for additional information on page 12.)*

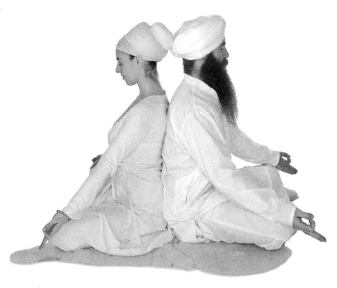

TIME: Chant the mantra out loud for **5 minutes**. Whisper the mantra for **5 minutes**. Meditate silently on the mantra for **10 minutes**. Whisper the mantra again for **5 minutes**. Chant the mantra out loud for **5 minutes**.

TO END: End with one minute of complete silence and stillness. Then, inhale and stretch the arms above the head, stretching the fingers wide. Stretch your spine and take several deep breaths, and relax.

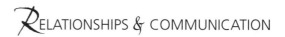

SHAKTI & SHAKTA: ONE HEART MEDITATION

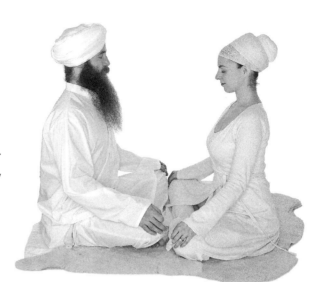

POSTURE: Sit down with your partner in any comfortable meditative position that maintain's a straight spine.

MUDRA: Relax arms and hands down in a comfortable position.

EYE FOCUS: Eyes can be closed half way, 9/10, or completely.

MANTRA & BREATH PATTERN: The mantra is the Mul Mantra. Take turns chanting the mantra. While your partner is chanting, hold the breath out.

Ek Ong Kaar, Sat Naam, Kartaa Purakh,
Nirbho, Nirvair, Akaal Moorat, Ajoonee,
Saibhang, Gur Prasaad, Jap.
Aad Sach, Jugaad Sach, Hai Bhee Sach, Naanak Hosee Bhee Sach

TIME: Build up to **31 minutes**. You may experience a sensation of weightlessness for about 10-15 minutes after completing the meditation.

About This Meditation

"When you chant he holds, and when he chants you hold. It is a good way for a husband and wife to relate to each other. The man should look like a man of God, and think a good thought. Woman is the symbol of Shakti, that which comes from the Infinite, is self-created, and which stands behind. Shakta, that which takes the Infinite and stands in front. One is Shakti and one Shakta—both are the polarity of the same divine force called God. Nobody is superior, nobody is inferior. One is the base and pushes up. The other gets pushed up from the base. So there are not two different things. That is why the grace of God is in you as a male or as a female. It is your moral strength. That is your honor, and that is why we feel it is a good thing for a person to live in his heart, not his head. Head is beautiful, head is not wrong—but something is beyond the head, and that is the heart, the Self, the being which throb's for somebody, which move's for something, which move's even when you don't move. Something which lives in you, when you feel you are dead, is your heart. The brain can collapse and revive, but when the heart collapses and it doesn't revive, the brain won't even function. The value of the Heart Chakra is very definite."

— Yogi Bhajan

This powerful couples' meditation is very invigorating, very energizing. It will give you a lot of strength and endurance. You can feel very light, because all of the functions become so tuned-in and effective. It restores you to a state of youthfulness and a time when everything was working perfectly. Holding the breath out flushes and purifies the blood. This is excellent for ridding the body of disease. Not only is it purifying for the blood, but it has the power to absorb oxygen so that the main functions of the body's organs gain a special kind of strength.

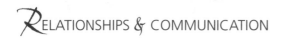

MANIFESTING GOD: SOPURKH

AUGUST 13, 1978

Shabd Guru

"Once, a man reached the stage of Guru because he gave the formula for acquiring infinite wealth within the values of the finite domain of human life. His contact with God was so beautiful that he recited this shabd, So Purkh:

ਸੋ ਪੁਰਖੁ ਨਿਰੰਜਨੁ ਹਰਿ ਪੁਰਖੁ ਨਿਰੰਜਨੁ
ਹਰਿ ਅਗਮਾ ਅਗਮ ਅਪਾਰਾ

*So purkh niranjan har purkh niranjan
har agamaa agam apaaraa.
That primal being is pure, that ever existent,
God, is immaculate.
He is endless and incomprehensible.*

–GURU RAM DAS, SIRI GURU GRANTH SAHIB, PAGE 10

You might sing this shabd as Gurbani, because for you it is Gurbani; but if you can perfect this shabd, God can appear before you, just as you can command a person into your presence. The vibratory effect of this shabd is so powerful, so par-excellent that the Par-Excellent and Yonder Excellence of the Excellent can manifest in person, in the shape of a man, in the presence of the one who has perfected this shabd. There are many beautiful shabds in the Siri Guru Granth Sahib, which are very powerful. Well, they're all powerful, but we do not illustratively know the powers of certain shabds. But we do know about So Purkh. So Purkh is the one shabd, chanted by Guru Ram Das, through which a person can manifest the Almighty, Omnipresent, Omniscient God—in personality—in one's own presence!"

—Yogi Bhajan

Recommendations for Practice

Yogi Bhajan taught women to recite *Sopurkh* 11 times a day to achieve mastery and to manifest God in their presence. It was recommended that women recite it as a prayer for the men in their lives. One recitation covers up to three men in your life at a time, for example, your father, your husband and your son. You can commit to 40 days, 90 days, 120 days, 1,000 days—or every day. You can recite it 11 times over the course of a week or a month. The most important thing is to keep building a relationship with this sound current. This practice is a powerful way to pray for the men in your life, clear your own karmas around men, and manifest the highest caliber of man to serve with you and your shared destiny.

For women in committed relationships, it's recommended to have this *shabd* playing at all times, but especially when your husband or partner is going through a hard time or if communication between the two of you is breaking down. For single women approaching this mantra, however, don't be mistaken. Your karmas must clear first. So for some it may feel like God is manifesting in the form of a Devil; that is, the same man you've been attracting your entire life! Have patience, continue to practice, and release yourself from any grasping. It is a pure prayer—and the prayer of a woman is always received and answered.

There are several audio versions available to support your practice; although Yogi Bhajan always recommended that you record your own voice and work with your own sound current. You will find the *Sopurkh shabd* in the *bani Rehiras*. See the resources page for more information.

SAT PURKH KAUR KHALSA
ESPAÑOLA, NEW MEXICO

Becoming a Mother

9 MONTHS, 40 DAYS & EVERYDAY

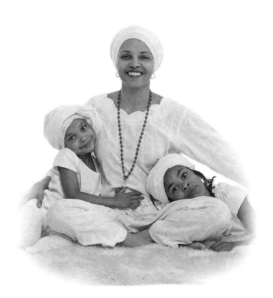

WHEN THE CHILD IS IN THE WOMB the frequency and strength of your nervous system will determine the health and vitality of the child's mental, physical and spiritual bodies. Your prayer will attract the soul that enters your being. The decision and the commitment to become a vessel for a new life is a most sacred act.

THE PRINCIPLE AND THE POWER OF THE MOTHER is within every woman, because whether she has children or not, she gives birth to creation after creation; bearing a child simply awakens this primal power of transformation. Being a mother is the most powerful creative act you can undertake. The sacrifice involved and the journey your soul takes with this child can never be understood until you've done it. As a mother you can create an angel or a demon. When the child is in the womb the frequency and strength of your nervous system will determine the health and vitality of the child's mental, physical and spiritual bodies. Your prayer will attract the soul that enters your being; therefore, the decision and the commitment to become a vessel for a new life is a most sacred act.

Becoming a mother is a journey and along the way you confront things within yourself you never thought you would, that in fact you didn't even know were there—and no one can truly prepare you for it. You are the child's first teacher, and for the first three years of her life, your aura and the child's auric field are one. From the first day of the child's life your life, your rhythm, even your waking and sleeping hours are no longer decided by you. The challenges you face are real. At times you are tested on every level—emotionally, physically and mentally. Yet at the same time you experience an overwhelming sense of devotion and unconditional love. Imagine this innocent child looking so lovingly at you—you! This is the beginning of a long journey, the greatest journey you will ever take in your life.

Because the act of becoming a mother is so profound and challenging—emotionally and spiritually—it's essential to prepare yourself on every level. For the first 40 days after childbirth your body is going through an incredible adjustment. It is a vital time to nurture yourself so that you can be revitalized and rebalanced. For the child it is a vital time to bond. This child is learning how to be at home on the Earth. If you are relaxed, contained and content, the child will be able to move forward in fearlessness and strength. Take care of you and keep the child in a serene environment so that the essential bonding of mother and child can be created. Many traumas in a child's life can be avoided if you make the time for this precious union now, in these first few weeks.

After the 40 days, the child continues to need a mother who gives values and virtues, creates a nurturing and caring environment, and brings a steady, calm hand and heart. Being present, deep listening and dedication to creating a future generation of givers and saints takes a great deal of commitment. In this chapter there are many techniques which will deliver you to victory. Remember to keep your discipline strong and most importantly be patient with yourself and the greatest creation you will ever experience, your child.

THE MEDITATIONS INCLUDED in this chapter lay the foundation for becoming a mother and give you the tools for the journey. A simple profound gift of Kundalini Yoga is meditation on the sound current, the pervasive pulse of spirit, which elevates both you and the child into the ecstasy of being human and being divine—together. To prepare for the journey, combine the practices of **Long Ek Ong Kar**, the *shabd*, ***Puta Mata Ki Asis***, and ***Charan Japa***. These techniques perfect the aura of the mother and the child and create a stable foundation for Infinity. **Long Ek Ong Kar** is also something that you should keep in your mother's kit for later in your child's life: practiced for 62 minutes a day it is said to cover the life of the child and protect her from harm, especially when it's self-inflicted.

The other meditations in this chapter build vitality and energy so that you have the stamina to keep up with your children, the strength and courage, in the face of extreme demands and fatigue, to keep going, and to constantly bring you back to your own divinity, your own grace, as the Adi Shakti—the Great Mother.

Becoming a mother is the greatest sacrifice and the greatest blessing. May these practices enable you to bring to the world a new generation of leaders, healers, and stewards of the planet, who bless the Aquarian Age with the gift of your creativity, your devotion and your divinity.

SAT PURKH KAUR KHALSA
& PRITPAL KAUR KHALSA
ESPAÑOLA, NEW MEXICO

LONG EK ONG KAR
LONG CHANT

POSTURE: Sit in Easy Pose with a firm Neck Lock.

MUDRA: Have the hands in Gyan Mudra, or resting in Buddha Mudra in the lap. Maintain a strong Neck Lock.

MANTRA: Chant the Adi Shakti Mantra in a 2-1/2 breath cycle:

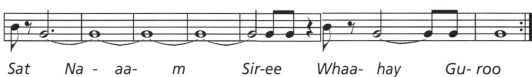

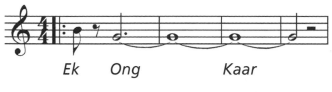

Ek   Ong   Kaar

Sat   Na - aa-   m   Sir-ee   Whaa- hay   Gu- roo

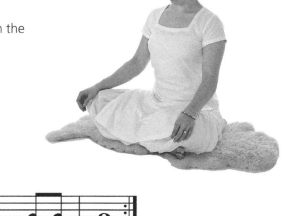

Inhale deeply and as you pull in the navel abruptly, chant *EK*. Then *ONG KAAR* is drawn out. Equal time to *ONG* and *KAAR*.
Inhale deeply and as you pull in the navel abruptly, chant *SAT*. Then *NAAM* is drawn out.
Then, just as you get to the end of the breath, add a quick SIREE. (pronounced S'ree.)
Inhale half a breath, pull in the navel abruptly, chant *WHAA*. Then *HAY GUROO* (*HAY* should be relatively short, *GUROO* is pronounced *G'ROO* and is drawn out, but not too long.
The *ONG KAAR* and *NAAM SIREE* are equal in length. The *WHAA-HAY GUROO* is equal in length to *ONG*.
Try not to let the pitch fall. Let the sound resonate in the upper cavity of the head, by closing the back of the throat and vibrating the upper palate, and allowing the sound to come through the nose.

TIME: 3-11 minutes. For a powerful experience of this meditation, do **31 minutes**, or **2-1/2 hours**.

About This Meditation

Yogi Bhajan speaks about this mantra: *"This mantra is known as the Ashtang Mantra for the Aquarian Age. It has eight vibrations, and describes the glory of God. Thus said the Master, 'In the time period two-and-a-half hours before the rising of the Sun, when the channels are most clear, if the Mantra is sung in sweet harmony, you will be one with the Lord.' This will open the solar plexus, which in turn will charge the solar centers, and the person will get connected with the Cosmic Energy, and thus will be liberated from the cycle of time and karma. Those who meditate on this mantra in silence will charge their solar centers and be one with the Divine. That is why I speak to you of why we should meditate and recite this mantra.*

"All mantras are good, and are for the awakening of the Divine. But this mantra is effective, and is the mantra for this Era. So my lovely student, at the will of my Master I teach you the greatest Divine key. It has eight levers, and can open the lock of the time, which is also of the vibration of eight. Therefore, when this mantra is chanted with the Neck Lock, at the point where prana and apana meet sushmuna, this vibration opens the lock, and thus one becomes one with the Divine."

This mantra is used as the cornerstone of morning sadhana, and is also called Long Ek Ong Kaar's or just Long Chant. This mantra initiates the kundalini, initiating the relationship between the soul and the Universal Soul. It balances all of the chakras. Though it is part of morning sadhana, it can be chanted at any time.

CHARAN JAPA AND BREATHWALK®
FLOURISHING THE SOUL OF A CHILD

POSTURE: Walking.

MUDRA, MANTRA & MOVEMENT: Man and woman, woman on the left, man on the right. His left hand, and her right hand are locked. Coordinate the steps with each other: on the left foot chant *SAT NAM*, on the right foot chant *WAHE GURU*.

TIME: 3-5 miles per day.

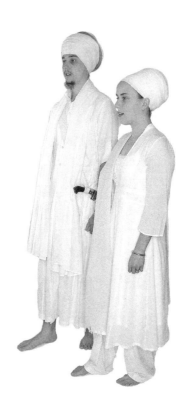

About This Meditation

This is called Charan Japa. It is an age-old method, in which a couple creates a rhythm and a frequency between them. It is very bonding and healing. It is especially beneficial if expecting a child. This bonded consciousness of the couple helps to flourish the soul of the child. This attracts a very easy, most beautiful child. The couple's own self is improved, too.

About Breathwalk® & Charan Japa

Yogi Bhajan shared with Gurucharan Singh Khalsa his approach to a simple, elegant walking technique based on the traditional system called Charan Japa or "repeat with the feet." A complete system called Breathwalk® was create, which goes beyond the basic traditonal *japa*, by integrating specific breath patterns, expanding the range of mantras, and including Kundalini Yoga exercises and guided meditation. In this way, one is able to direct mood, energy and awareness in multiple ways. It has been proven to be one of the most powerful physical exercises to break stress, improve health and gain emotional control. It is not only an accessible natural activity, but also a deep meditation and a profound way to connect to nature—inner and outer.

GUIDANCE KRIYA

JULY 11, 1986

POSTURE: Sit in Easy Pose with the spine straight, and a light Neck Lock.

EYE FOCUS: Eyes are closed.

MANTRA & MOVEMENT:
Meditate to a musical recording of *Rakhe Rakhanhar* and move in this way:

(1) Bring the arms up and hold opposite forearms near the elbows. Inhale in **8 strokes**, gently swinging the arms from side-to-side in rhythm with the breath and to the beat of the music (as if rocking a baby).

(2) Exhale, and lower the arms to rest on the knees in Gyan Mudra.

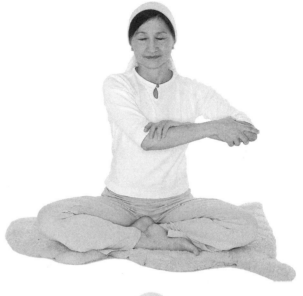

Rakhay rakhanhaar aap ubaarian
Gur kee pairee paa-eh kaaj savaarian
Hoaa aap dayaal manho na visaarian
Saadh janaa kai sung bhavjal taarian
Saakat nindak dusht khin maa-eh bidaarian
Tis saahib kee tayk naanak manai maa-eh
Jis simrat sukh ho-eh saglay dookh jaa-eh

Continue inhaling and exhaling and moving in this way to the music at your own pace.

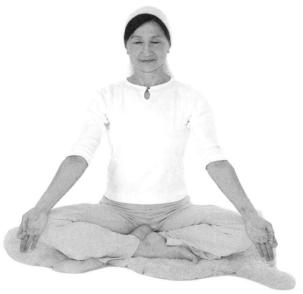

TIME: 31 minutes.

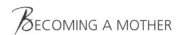
MEDITATION FOR **TREMENDOUS STRENGTH**

NOVEMBER 2, 1978

POSTURE: Sit in Easy Pose with a straight spine, and a light Neck Lock.

PART ONE

MUDRA: Relax arms down with the hands resting on the knees.

EYE FOCUS: The eyes are closed.

BREATH: Breathe in long, deep, slow complete breaths. Make the breath as long and slow as possible.

MANTRA: There is no mantra for this portion of the meditation. If available, the gong can be played. Ride on the sound current of the infinite. Either totally relax in the deepest meditation possible or be totally tense and come apart as the gong is played. Do not drink any water for 30 minutes after you have listened to the gong.

TIME: 11 minutes.

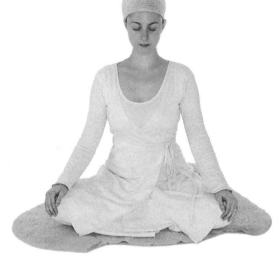

About Part One

The sympathetic nervous system is operated by the principles of light. The parasympathetic nervous system is operated by the principle of sound. The muscular system operates by the gross Earth. In the supreme combination of human psychology, the greatest strength lies in the parasympathetic nervous system. The music of the gong, which is the sound of the infinite, can heal this system.

PART TWO

MUDRA: Draw the forearms up until the hands meet at the level of the throat, palms facing each other, fingers pointing up. Separate the fingers and thumb of each hand. Press the corresponding fingertip of the opposite hands forming a tepee-like structure. The thumbs do not touch at all, and the Saturn (middle) and Jupiter (index) fingers maintain only light contact. Apply maximum pressure on the Mercury (pinkie) and Sun (ring) fingers.

EYE FOCUS: Closed.

BREATH: Breathe very slowly, very long, and very deep. Focus on the various pressures on the different fingers and on the long, slow, deep breathing. Concentrate very deeply.

TIME: 8 minutes.

TO END: Deeply inhale and stretch the arms high over the head. Hold the breath in and stretch as hard as possible. Completely exhale and leave the hands up. Deeply inhale, hold, and stretch. Completely exhale and relax.

About Part Two

This part of the meditation will bring you an experience of tremendous strength and can trigger new life in you. By putting more pressure on the Sun and Mercury fingers a balance is created in the Id by the action of the earth into the parasympathetic nervous system. For the first 3-5 minutes nothing but irritation will be experienced. If you can go through it, a relaxation never before experienced will come. The meditation alters the superconscious present in everyday consciousness. A simple self-created magnetic field, with a polarity opposite to the normal function is created. If the breath is controlled, meditated upon, and kept long and slow enough it will not enter the diaphragm. The 8th vertabra will start secreting. The impulsation of the pituitary gland will then change.

PART THREE

MUDRA: Bring the right hand on top of the left, palms down, at the Heart Center. The elbows are extended to each side. The fingers of each hand are together but the thumbs are extended toward the chest. Bend the wrists so that the elbows are slightly higher than the hands.

EYE FOCUS: Eyes are closed.

MANTRA: Chant the Kundalini Shakti mantra in a monotone voice as the breath is completely exhaled from the lungs.

AAD SACH, JUGAAD SACH, HAI BHEE SACH
NAANAK HOSEE BHEE SACH

TIME: Continue for **31 minutes**.

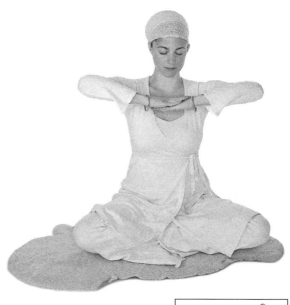

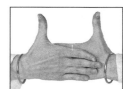

About Part Three

Man has the power of the word in the power of sound. The hypothalamus rests on the upper palate of the mouth, which has 84 meridian points. When these meridian points are struck by the tongue, the hypothalamus circulates in rhythm with the circulation of the impulsation of the pituitary and pineal glands. This rhythm causes the glandular system secretions to match up with the impulsations in the magnetic field of the body, and bridge the gaps when this field is weak. When a rhythm of 60 impulsations per second is reached, a rebuilding process in the magnetic field and in the life is triggered and an experience of Infinity may be the result.

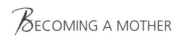

MEDITATION TO **KEEP UP WITH OUR CHILDREN**
JANUARY 23, 1973

POSTURE: Sit in Easy Pose with a straight spine, and a light Neck Lock.

MUDRA: Touch the tips of the thumb and the Jupiter (index) fingers. The remaining fingers are folded into the palm.

EYE FOCUS: Eyes are focused at the solar center (top of the head).

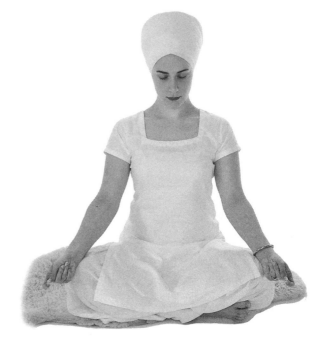

PART ONE
MANTRA: Inhale, concentrating on the solar center while mentally projecting:

> *SAA TAA*

Exhale as you mentally project:

> *NAA MAA*

TIME: 31 minutes.

PART TWO
Bring the chin up. Chant the *Sat Nam Wahe Guru* mantra in a monotone, with a steady, rapid rhythm:

> *SAT NAAM SAT NAAM SAT NAAM SAT NAAM*
> *SAT NAAM SAT NAAM WHAA-HAY GUROO*

TIME: 5-7 minutes.

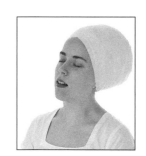

About This Meditation

This meditation will help you handle the more sensitive brain activity needed for the coming Era, and allows you to keep up with your children.

"The human race is getting into a very mentally sensitive era. The new generation is nothing but a bunch of vibrations. People are going to become more and more sensitive and not understand why they feel the way they do. Ninety percent of people will go crazy. Astrologically, because of the influence of Uranus, we are experiencing more sensitive brain activity. The mental projection is becoming more activated; controlling and channeling it will be a problem; out-of-body experiences will be almost uncontrollable. And the children being born and raised now are much more sensitive than we were as children. By the time we are 50-60 years old we will not be able to understand the children at all, the gap will be so wide." —Yogi Bhajan

MEDITATION ON THE **DIVINE MOTHER** ADI SHAKTI

NOVEMBER 16, 1973

PART ONE

POSTURE: Sit in Easy Pose, the hands in Gyan Mudra.

EYE FOCUS: Eyes are closed.

VISUALIZATION: Meditate on the Infinite energy coming from the primal womb, in an unending spiral, without beginning or end, going to Infinity. Visualize the *yantra* (symbolic form) in the eight-wheel form.

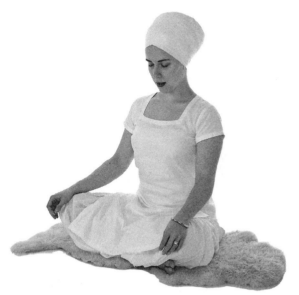

PART TWO

With the eyes closed, cup the hands with palms 4-6 inches (10-15 cm) apart, in front of the face. Beam a mental light through them to the Infinite Light. Watch with mental eyes, through the hands, and see a beam of light going to Infinity. This is very mind-curing, and you will fall in love with it. Meditate with Long Deep Breathing.

PART THREE

Mentally chant the Panj Shabd: *SAA TAA NAA MAA*. Go deeper into meditation. Guide your reason to go through the powerful imaginative circle you've created with your hands, like a huge beam of light from a torch. Keep the hands fixed in place.

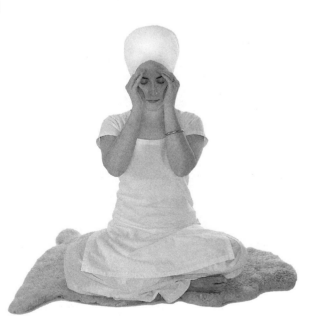

meditation continues on next page

PART FOUR

Maintain your position and concentration. Put your mind into that Infinite Light of its own ecstasy and chant the Kundalini Bhakti Mantra.

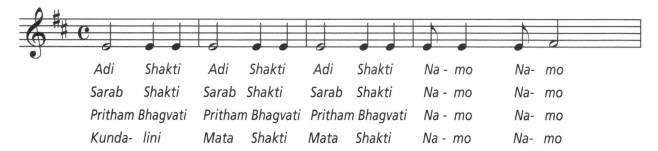

Adi	Shakti	Adi	Shakti	Adi	Shakti	Na - mo	Na- mo
Sarab	Shakti	Sarab	Shakti	Sarab	Shakti	Na - mo	Na- mo
Pritham Bhagvati		Pritham Bhagvati		Pritham Bhagvati		Na - mo	Na- mo
Kunda- lini		Mata	Shakti	Mata	Shakti	Na - mo	Na- mo

I bow to the Primal Power.
I bow to the all Encompassing Power and Energy.
I bow to that through which God creates.
I bow to the creative power of the kundalini, the Divine Mother Power.

TIME: All four parts of this meditation should be done for equal lengths of time. 11, 31, or 62 minutes each.

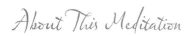

About This Meditation

This meditation gives concentration and mental beaming. It tunes into the frequency of the Divine Mother—the primal, protective, generating energy. It eliminates fears and fulfills desires. It empowers you to act by removing blocks and insecurity.

　"Let us call on the Divine Mother, the Infinite, the Powerful. Let us talk to her. You will require a little mental imagination. If she is not with you, create it! Her yantra (symbolic form) is the two swords of God to protect you, the center of your world. These are the two-edged swords of the being—the negative and positive. This is her being, this is her presence. We have to use the faculty of our imagination on and through something. This is Infinity within us."　—Yogi Bhajan

THE **MOTHER'S PRAYER**
PUTA MATA KI ASIS

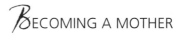
Shabd Guru

EVERY WOMAN EMBODIES THE ENERGY of the Kundalini Mata Shakti: The Creative Power of the Mother. When a woman decides to assist a soul in coming to the planet in human form, it is a tremendous responsibility. In *Japji Sahib*, Guru Nanak said that the human birth is very rare and very precious, for it is only in the human body that the Tenth Gate, the door of liberation, can be found. A soul can only incarnate into human form if it has earned that privilege in its previous births, and if it has been blessed with grace. So when a woman conceives a child, she becomes the channel of divine opportunity for a worthy and deserving soul; and she can use her creative power to awaken—her identity as Mata Shakti—to bless her own child through her prayer.

Because the mother is the first teacher, and those lessons begin in the womb, the consciousness of the mother is tremendously important. Every word a woman says during her pregnancy, every thought, every feeling, every experience provides the foundation, the vibration from which the body of the child is formed. It is natural for a woman to imagine what she wants and hopes for her child. That desire, good or bad, has an impact on the sensitive soul-consciousness that is meditating and developing in her womb.

To help a woman hold the highest intention and prayer for her child, Guru Arjan, the fifth Sikh Master, composed the *shabd*, *Puta Mata Ki Asis*. This *shabd* embodies the purest prayer that a mother can wish for her child. Subconsciously, this *shabd* helps the woman and the child understand the purpose of their relationship to one another. The purpose of the mother is to serve and support the soul of the child so that it has a chance to attain liberation in this lifetime. The purpose of the child is to understand this chance and do her best to fulfill it. Any other relationship between the mother and child is maya, a worldly trap. If the relationship becomes one of ego and too much attachment, both the mother and the child create karma for themselves. If the relationship is one of projective prayer on the part of the mother for the highest spiritual destiny of her child; and if the child can receive that prayer and deliver it—both are liberated. Not only that, when a child reaches the state that is described in this *shabd*, seven generations before and after attain liberation as well. What higher hope and prayer can there be for one's baby?

This *shabd* talks about the beauty of a life spent devoted to meditation on the Divine. It talks of deep peace, love and happiness. As a mother vibrates, so the core identity of her child becomes. When this *shabd* is offered as a prayer, and sung without ego, attachment or desire, in total surrender to the Divine, especially while the child is preparing to come into the world, during pregnancy, it gives the soul of that child that much more of a chance to realize its destiny and become liberated—merging into the experience of oneness with the Divine.

EK ONG KAAR KAUR KHALSA
ESPAÑOLA, NEW MEXICO

ਪੂਤਾ ਮਾਤਾ ਕੀ ਆਸੀਸ
ਨਿਮਖ ਨ ਬਿਸਰਉ ਤੁਮ੍ ਕਉ ਹਰਿ ਹਰਿ ਸਦਾ ਭਜਹੁ ਜਗਦੀਸ

THE MOTHER'S PRAYER
PUTA MATA KI ASIS
Guru Arjan Dev, Siri Guru Granth Sahib, page 496

ਗੂਜਰੀ ਮਹਲਾ 5
ਜਿਸੁ ਸਿਮਰਤ ਸਭਿ ਕਿਲਵਿਖ ਨਾਸਹਿ ਪਿਤਰੀ ਹੋਇ ਉਧਾਰੋ
ਸੋ ਹਰਿ ਹਰਿ ਤੁਮ੍ ਸਦ ਹੀ ਜਾਪਹੁ ਜਾ ਕਾ ਅੰਤੁ ਨ ਪਾਰੋ ॥1॥

ਪੂਤਾ ਮਾਤਾ ਕੀ ਆਸੀਸ ॥ ਨਿਮਖ ਨ ਬਿਸਰਉ ਤੁਮ੍ ਕਉ ਹਰਿ ਹਰਿ
ਸਦਾ ਭਜਹੁ ਜਗਦੀਸ ॥1॥ ਰਹਾਉ ॥
ਸਤਿਗੁਰੁ ਤੁਮ੍ ਕਉ ਹੋਇ ਦਇਆਲਾ ਸੰਤਸੰਗਿ ਤੇਰੀ ਪ੍ਰੀਤਿ
ਕਾਪੜੁ ਪਤਿ ਪਰਮੇਸਰੁ ਰਾਖੀ ਭੋਜਨੁ ਕੀਰਤਨੁ ਨੀਤਿ ॥2॥

ਅੰਮ੍ਰਿਤੁ ਪੀਵਹੁ ਸਦਾ ਚਿਰੁ ਜੀਵਹੁ ਹਰਿ ਸਿਮਰਤ ਅਨਦ ਅਨੰਤਾ
ਰੰਗ ਤਮਾਸਾ ਪੂਰਨ ਆਸਾ ਕਬਹਿ ਨ ਬਿਆਪੈ ਚਿੰਤਾ ॥3॥
ਭਵਰੁ ਤੁਮਾਰਾ ਇਹੁ ਮਨੁ ਹੋਵਉ ਹਰਿ ਚਰਣਾ ਹੋਹੁ ਕਉਲਾ
ਨਾਨਕ ਦਾਸੁ ਉਨਿ ਸੰਗਿ ਲਪਟਾਇਓ ਜਿਉ ਬੂੰਦਹਿ ਚਾਤ੍ਰਿਕੁ ਮਉਲਾ ॥4॥3॥4॥

Gujri Mahalaa 5
Jis simrat sabh kilvikh naaseh pitree ho-eh odaaro
So har har tum sad hee jaapho jaa kaa ant na paaro
Putaa maataa kee aasees nimakh na bisaro tum kau har har.
Sadaa bhajho jagdees (Rahaau)
Satgur tum kau hoeh dyaalaa santsang tayree preet
Kaapar(d) pat parmaysar raakhee bhojan keertan neet
Amrit peevho sadaa chir jeevho har simrat anad anant
Rang tamaasaa pooran aasaa kabeh na biaapai chintaa
Bhavar tumaaraa eho man hovau har charnaa ho-ho kaulaa
Nanak daas on sang laptaaio jeeo boondeh chaatrik maulaa

RAAG GUJRI, FIFTH CHANNEL OF LIGHT
Remembering Him, all sins are erased, and ones generations are saved.
So meditate continually on the Lord, Har, Har; He has no end or limitation. ॥ 1 ॥
O child, this is your mother's blessing, that you may never forget the Lord, Har, Har, even for an instant.
May you ever vibrate the Lord of the Universe. ॥ 1 ॥ Pause ॥
May the True Guru be kind to you, and may you love the Society of the Saints.
May the preservation of your honor by the Transcendent Lord be your clothing,
and may the singing of His Praises be your food. ॥ 2 ॥
So drink in forever the Ambrosial Nectar. May you live long, may the meditative remembrance of the Lord give you
infinite delight. May joy and pleasure be yours. May your hopes be fulfilled, and may you never be troubled by worries. ॥ 3 ॥
Let this mind of yours be the bumble bee, and let the Lord's feet be the lotus flower. Says servant Nanak,
attach your mind to them, and blossom forth like the songbird, upon finding the raindrop. ॥ 4 ॥ 3 ॥ 4 ॥

TRANSFORMATIONS & TRANSITIONS

BREATHING THROUGH EVERYTHING

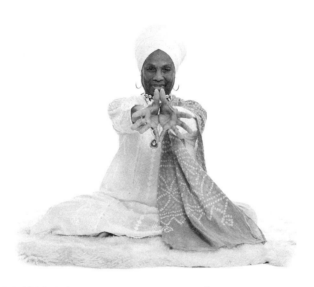

MAY YOU NEVER BE AFRAID of your own excellence. With every breath you have the opportunity to change, to transform. Use the breath to elevate yourself to that highest destiny, and allow the breath to carry you across any and every obstacle.

THE BREATH, PRANA, IS THE KEY TO LIFE, for without it there is no life; it's also the key to your best life, your excellence. Breath control can become your greatest ally and friend. Breath is the key to balancing your hormones, your emotions, and can even help you negotiate—and win. If you can breathe slower than your counterpart, you'll always come out ahead. Breath is a discipline and a flow. It is a wave, a vibration, carrying with it a sound current that confirms and reaffirms your divinity—*sohung*—inhale, *so*, exhale *hung*. "*I am that; I am the breath of life.*" And in this way you merge in the identity of God.

Mastering your breath is important throughout your life, but in those key moments of transition and transformation, it can be the vehicle that literally and figuratively carries you across that vast ocean of consciousness, changing roles and identities, and ultimately death. Using the breath to serve you and your consciousness is the key to vitality—and if you also have a touch of grace, it can be the key to a 'good death.'

Five Pranayam Techniques

This chapter opens with five *pranayam* techniques. Being familiar with them will help you in your practice of other kriyas, but their mastery alone can take you anywhere you want to go.

One Minute Breath allows you to still your mind, practice silence and begin to hear a deeper sound current. It also builds the Radiant Body and disciplines speech by cultivating patience. Guru Gobind Singh was said to have mastered this breath—and even in battle maintained this discipline. He and Yogi Bhajan both explained in detail how woman can use her power to create or destroy. By mastering her breath, woman can master her moods and her reactions so she can go beyond her weaknesses to meet life's challenges successfully. In this way, she can create an absolute Heaven on Earth, instead of the hell that comes when her emotions are in charge.

Breath of Fire, as its name implies, strengths your inner fire and builds the *agni*. It purifies, cleanses, and heals. Yogi Bhajan said that 31 minutes a day of Breath of Fire could heal anything, and could literally, "save the day."

Sitali Pranayam is a cooling breath, excellent for calming the heart and mind, and bringing a 'moon-like' quality into the body. Twenty-five repetitions in the morning and in the evening can balance the hormonal body, especially during the body's major transitions: menstrual cycle and menopause.

Segmented breathing, or **Four Stroke Breath**, creates balance and discipline. The simple rhythm of the segmented breath, especially when combined with a mental mantra, such as the Panj Shabd (*Sa Ta Na Ma*), not only builds vitality but also generates an imprint of that healing sound current within the mind and body's rhythm.

Alternate Nostril Breathing, too, is a balancing breath. With the inhale on the left, calming and cooling qualities ride on the breath; and the breath in the right nostril brings in energy, fire, and strength.

Learn to use these various pranayams—master them—so that you direct the mind's flow with the breath. There are other practices in this chapter that are specific to various life cycles and transitions. Apply them as necessary and experience a newfound balance and equanimity in the face of transformation and change. Yogi Bhajan loved to create pressure and challenge for his students, because facing the tests and changes of life requires us to reach deep, and truly realize our strength beyond what we might normally volunteer.

One final note, the two *shabd* practices, the *Pran Sutra* and *Anand Sahib*, are critical to mastering life's transformations and transitions. Yogi Bhajan emphasized practicing the *pran shabd* any time you faced insecurity or doubt throughout the day; so that when you came to that final hour—that final breath—you would have already imprinted this sound current in your mind. And with that last breath this sound current carries you across any fear, or anxiety.

In the same way, the *Anand Sahib* can serve you in making it through the transitions in your life, helping to heal any gaps, and integrate the self and the soul with the life's course. *Anand Sahib* allows you to live in the flow, trust in the good, and reside in bliss.

In teaching *shabd*, Yogi Bhajan explained that the ultimate goal for woman is to embed the infinite sound current, which cuts away our ego, into the core of our being while we are young. This allows us to vibrate in such a state of inner stillness that we can listen with our whole brain to our Truth, our intuition, our inner Infinity. Then when it is time for us to transition through menopause into our later years, this skill will give us the vitality and altitude to keep our balance so that we truly can become wise, sacred women as we age, and avoid taking on the quali-

ties of a man (because of the decrease in estrogen). When we can unite our breath with mantra or *shabd*, our breath becomes our teacher, building our inner guidance and sensitivity so that we can act in integrity, without doubt.

May you never be afraid of your own excellence. Know that with every breath you have the chance, the opportunity to change, to transform. Use the breath to elevate yourself to that highest destiny, and allow the breath to carry you across any and every obstacle.

DEVA KAUR KHALSA
CORAL SPRINGS, FLORIDA

SAT PURKH KAUR KHALSA
ESPAÑOLA, NEW MEXICO

THE BREATH OF LIFE: FIVE BASIC PRANAYAMS

The quantity, quality, and circulation of the breath creates the foundation of a vital and creative life. It is a barometer of how much energy we normally run on, and how much reserve capacity we have created for emergencies. The breath is both gross and subtle. The gross aspect is the blend of oxygen, nitrogen, and other elements that constitute air. The subtle aspect is the *prana* or vital force that energizes the mind, body, and consciousness.

Most people do not breath correctly. Breath signatures that create shallow, erratic, upper-chest breathing are common. The lack of relaxation and well-being on a personal as well as collective level, along with other factors, inhibits proper breathing. Yet, of all the positive changes a person can make, learning to breathe deeply, and completely is probably the most effective for developing higher consciousness, and for increasing health, vitality, and connectedness in one's life.

Here are five basic yogic breaths that can give you new life. Make them part of your life.

ALTERNATE NOSTRIL BREATHING

POSTURE: Sit in a comfortable position.

MUDRA & BREATH:
In this *pranayam*, the breath is always relaxed, deep and full. Have the left hand in Gyan Mudra. Use the thumb of the right hand to close the right nostril, and the index finger or ring finger of the right hand to close the left nostril.

Close one nostril and slowly, deeply and fully inhale through that nostril. Then close the opposite nostril and slowly, deeply and fully exhale, bringing the navel towards the spine.

Continue this pattern.

Note: Inhaling left, exhaling right: helps to make you calm and integrates unwanted negative emotions and stress. Excellent by itself before bed.

Inhaling right, exhaling left: gives clarity, and postive mood. Helps to focus on what is important.

TIME: Continue **3-31 minutes**.

TO END: Inhale through both nostrils, hold, exhale. Sit quietly and still.

About Alternate Nostril Breathing

This simple, yet most powerful technique, is a *pranayam* that is easy to do,
yet creates a deep sense of well-being and harmony on the physical, mental, and emotional levels. It is integrating and grounding, and induces the systemic functions of the entire brain by balancing the right and left hemispheres. Can be helpful in dealing with headaches, migraines, and other stress-related symptoms.

FOUR STROKE BREATH

POSTURE: Sit in a comfortable position.

BREATH: Inhale in four heavy strokes, then exhale in one long stroke.

EYE FOCUS: Focus at the tip of the nose.

TIME: 3-11 minutes.

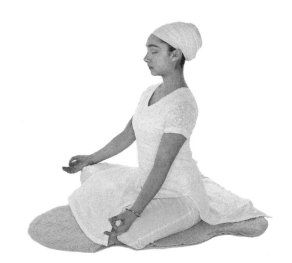

About Four Stroke Breath

This four-stroke segmented breath will open up your lung capacity to absorb more oxygen which you need for life. It will give you more patience, more tolerance. It gives you the capacity to develop a more effective breath pattern. On average, people breath 15 breaths per minute. If you want to have success in life, slow your breathing down to 5 breaths a minute. You live by breath. You die by breath.

SITALI PRANAYAM

POSTURE: Sit in a comfortable position.

BREATH: Close the eyes and concentrate at the Brow Point, the Third Eye Point. Roll your tongue into a "U" with the tip just outside the lips. If you cannot roll your tongue, stick the tip outside the mouth and curve it. Inhale breathing through the rolled tongue. Exhale through the nose.

TIME: 3-11 minutes.

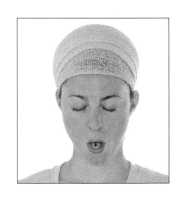

About Sitali Pranayam

Sitali Pranayam cools and relaxes. It is used often by yogis to clear the head and aid digestion. This *pranayam* can be very helpful during pregnancy to lessen heartburn. If your tongue tastes bitter when you practice Sitali, it is an indication of toxification. Continue practicing regularly for best results.

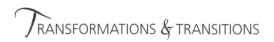

ONE MINUTE BREATH

POSTURE: Sit in Easy Pose with Neck Lock.

BREATH: Inhale very slowly for 20 seconds. Hold for 20 seconds, pull the spine up, drop the shoulders. Exhale very slowly for 20 seconds. Continue in that pattern.

TIME: Begin to practice for **3 minutes**, increase gradually up to **31 minutes**.

About One Minute Breath

This is a very effective, advanced pranayam.

"If you can breathe one breath a minute, you can overcome everything and anything you have to face in life. The One Minute Breath builds endurance, strengthens your lungs and diaphragm for birthing. You say you are depressed? What is "depressed"? Depressed is you have impressed yourself that God is not with you— that's depressed. What is "sad"? You are sad because you have not found the depth of your breath. When you are most sad, start breathing one breath a minute. If you are still sad on the fourth breath, call me!" —Yogi Bhajan

BREATH OF FIRE

- Breath of Fire is rapid, rhythmic, and continuous. It is equal on the inhale and the exhale, with no pause between them. (Approximately 2-3 cycles per second.)
- It is always practiced through the nostrils with mouth closed, unless stated otherwise.
- Breath of Fire is powered from the Navel Point and solar plexus. To exhale, the air is expelled through the nose, by pressing the Navel Point and solar plexus back toward the spine. This feels automatic if you contract the diaphragm rapidly.
- The inhale comes in as part of relaxation rather than through effort; the upper abdominal muscles relax, the diaphragm extends down, and the breath naturally comes in to fill the vacuum created by the exhale.
- The chest stays relaxed and slightly lifted throughout the breathing cycle.
- When done correctly, there should be no rigidity in the hands, feet, face, or abdomen.

TIME: Begin practicing for **1-3 minutes**. Gradually increase to **31 minutes**, or apply as needed to appropriate *kriyas*.

About Breath of Fire

Breath of Fire is one of the primary breath techniques used in the practice of Kundalini Yoga. It accompanies many postures, and has numerous beneficial effects. Mastery of this breath will give you great command of your Self and mastery over the Lower Triangle of Chakras. It purifies the blood, expands the lung capacity, and strengthens the nervous system to deal with stress.

Some people find it easy to do Breath of Fire for a full 10 minutes right away. Others find that the breath creates an initial dizziness or giddiness. If this happens, take a break. Some tingling, traveling sensations, and lightheadedness are completely normal as your body adjusts to the new breath and new stimulation of the nerves. Concentrating at the Brow Point may help relieve these sensations. Sometimes these symptoms are the result of toxins and other chemicals released by the breath technique. The symptoms may be relieved by drinking lots of water and changing to a light diet.

Breath of Fire while pregnant is not advised. Refrain from practicing Breath of Fire during the first or second days of your menstruation, depending on the intensity of the flow. In general, women are advised to increase their awareness of their bodies during menstruation and adapt the level of exercise accordingly. A light Breath of Fire is permissible during the rest of the menstrual cycle.

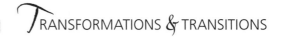

STAYING RELAXED AND BALANCED
THROUGH YOUR MOON TIME

The monthly cycle of menstruation is a major hormonal event. Estrogen levels can change greatly. As the chemical levels vary there are corresponding changes in emotions, a switch in the dominance of the brain hemispheres, and shifts in cognitive abilities—some improve and others lessen. For many women, menstruation is accompanied by cramps and pain. Sometimes this comes from too little exercise and a cumulative build-up of tension. The lack of movement and breathing stops the body from adjusting itself. Tension often builds up and registers in the ovaries, making them rigid and immobile. Normally. the ovaries go through a slow contraction and lifting motion during the month. If the tension is too high, this motion is interrupted. The body attempts to compensate with inappropriate muscles and nerves. This leads to pain and irregularities.

If you experience chronic problems with tension and/or menstruation, practice the following meditation and kriya every day for 40 days. During that time, eat a light diet, drink plenty of water and drink Yogi Tea.

BREATH RHYTHM TO **REGULATE THE MENSTRUAL CYCLE**

POSTURE: Sit in Easy Pose, with the spine straight.

MUDRA: Wrists are resting on the knees, elbows straight, palms facing up.

BREATH & MANTRA:
Inhale through the nose in a four-part Segmented Breath.

Press the index finger to the thumb on the first sniff,
as you mentally vibrate *SAA*.

Press the middle finger to the thumb on the second sniff,
as you mentally vibrate *TAA*.

Press the ring finger to the thumb on the third sniff,
as you mentally vibrate *NAA*.

Press the little finger to the thumb on the fourth sniff,
as you mentally vibrate *MAA*.

Exhale in one long stroke.
The rhythm will be 8 beats: Inhale segmented breath in 4 strokes, exhale in one long stroke for 4 beats.

EYE FOCUS: Eyes are closed.

TIME: Begin with 3 minutes. The time can be increased by 1 minute daily up to 7 minutes, then practiced for a week or so at 7 minutes, then increased again by a 1 minute per day, up to 31 minutes.

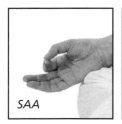 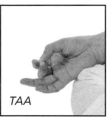 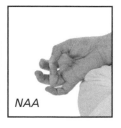 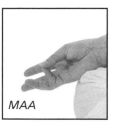

SAA   TAA   NAA   MAA

About This Pranayam

On the physical level, the pituitary and pineal glands are stimulated and brought into rhythm by the four part breathing. On a mental level, negative thought patterns can be erased and a new balance established. On an auric level, a clear radiance and projection can be achieved.

RELEASING MENSTRUAL TENSION *&* BALANCING SEXUAL ENERGY

1. Sit on the heels. Extend the left leg straight back along the ground. Bend forward and place the forehead on the ground. Put both arms back along the sides, palms up. Relax all the muscles and breath slowly and deeply. **3 minutes**. Then slowly rise up on the inhale. Repeat on the other side for **3 minutes**.

This exercise is a meditation itself. The time of practice can gradually be increased to 11 minutes on each side. It becomes a self-trance meditation. The pituitary gland is stimulated and the ovaries are relaxed. This posture is also excellent for the eyes.

2. **Throat & Neck Massage**. Sit on the heels. With one hand, gently massage the muscles on each side of the throat and neck. Use a wave-like motion from the collarbone up to the jaw. Continue this rhythmic squeeze for **2 minutes**.

This exercise is for the thyroid gland and Fifth Chakra.

3. **Ear Massage**. Still on the heels. Bring the heel of the hands to the ears, keeping the fingers together and pointed slightly behind you. Create a slight angle at the wrists so the fingers point away from the skull. Massage the ears and earlobes with the palms. Alternate between circular motion and linear up and down strokes. Continue for **2-3 minutes**. Inhale and gently pull the earlobes downward and away from the body. Hold for **10 seconds** and relax.

This is for lymphatic stimulation and circulation. There are meridian points on the ears that govern all parts of the body. It is a whole body massage using just the ears.

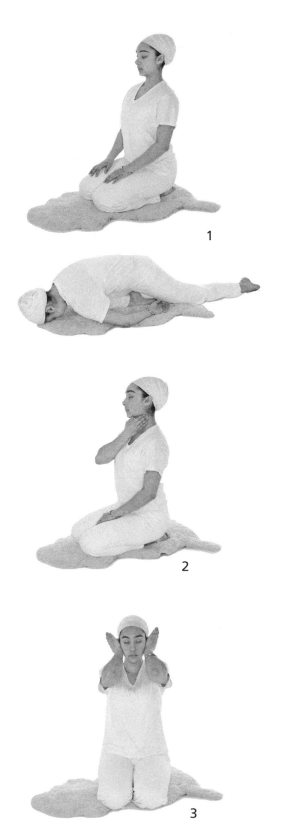

4. **Torso Twists**. Still sitting on the heels, immediately interlace the fingers in Venus Lock at the base of the spine. Keep the spine straight. Inhale deeply as you twist the torso to the left. Exhale and turn to the right. The motion is moderately slow and complete. Continue for **3 minutes**. To end inhale, pull *mulbandh* and concentrate on the full length of the spine. Imagine energy flowing up the center of the spine rejuvenating and relaxing the whole body. Exhale and relax.

This is for the lumbar spine and relaxation in the pelvis. It also helps elimination.

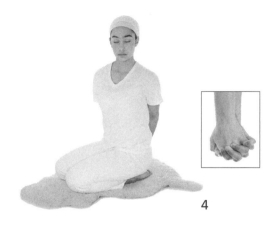

4

5. **Sit-ups with Legs Wide**. Lie on the back. Spread the legs as wide as possible, without strain. Grasp the shoulders, and let the elbows rest on the ground. Mentally survey all the muscles in the body.

Moving very slowly, muscle by muscle, bring the torso gradually up until you bend all the way forward, placing the forehead on the ground. Hold this position with relaxed breaths for **3 minutes**. Inhale deeply as you lie back and relax.

Gradually rise up and forward again. This time bend over the left knee. Hold the pose for **I minute**. Inhale and exhale deeply **3 times**. Then inhale deeply as you lie back.

Repeat the same sit-up and hold over the right leg. Hold for **I minute**. Inhale and exhale deeply **3 times**. Then inhale deeply as you lie back.

This is for the sciatic nerve and its branches. It strengthens the abdomen and lets go of tension caused by anxiety.

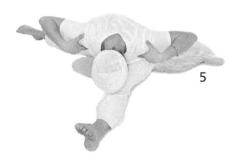

5

6. **Knee & Elbow Walk**. Balance on the hands and knees. Raise the heels toward the buttocks. Place the elbows on the ground, with the hands up by the shoulders. Raise the head so you can see forward. Begin to walk on elbows and knees. Continue for **3 minutes**. Relax completely on the back for **I minute**.

This promotes circulation, works on the heart, and improves the mineral balance.

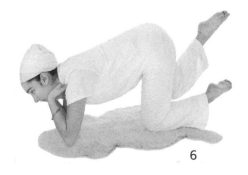

6

7. **Lotus Walk**. Sit in **Full Lotus Pose**. (Lock the feet on the upper thighs.) Put the hands on the ground beside the knees. Lean forward onto the hands and swing the body ahead. Repeat the motion so you scoot along the ground. Continue for **3 minutes**.

This opens the Navel Point energy, helps headaches and relaxes the sex organs.

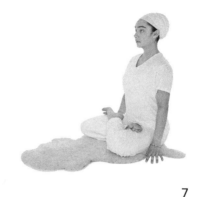

7

8. **Back Platform Pose**. Sit straight with the legs stretched out in front, toes pointed. Put the hands on the ground in back and lift the hips up until a straight platform is formed from the chin to the tip of the toes. Raise the head to look forward. Keep the legs straight and begin to "walk" on the heels and hands. Continue for **3 minutes**.

This releases mental anxiety and tension, and strengthens the lower back and hips.

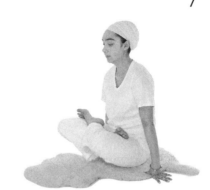

9. **Deep Relaxation**. Totally relax on the back. Become weightless and float into the blue ethers. **15 minutes**.

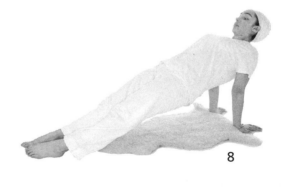

8

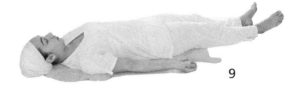

9

About This Kriya

This series adjusts the energy in the sex meridians. It releases the tension in the ovaries and enhances circulation to the pelvic region. It is also an excellent set for men: it balances the sexual energy and helps the prostate.

EMOTIONAL AND MENTAL BALANCE
AND PREVENTION OF EARLY MENOPAUSE
JULY 21, 1977

1. In a standing position with knees and heels together, feet are flat on the ground, with the big toes pointing out to the sides for balance. Arms are raised straight overhead, close to the ears with the palms facing forward. (The thumbs can be locked together.) Keeping the legs straight, bend back from the base of the spine 20 degrees. The head, spine and arms form an unbroken curve with the arms remaining in a line with the ears. Hold the posture and keep the breath long, deep and gentle. **2 minutes**.

This exercise is called "Miracle Bend." It doesn't bend the human being, it bends the negativity in the human being. It adjusts the Navel Point and helps bring an emotional and angry person to calmness. If the spine were bent to 90 degrees and the breath was four times per minute, it would also totally calm a person. But that takes a very long time, whereas this exercise takes only a short time. There will be a strong and automatic tendency to shake in the posture.

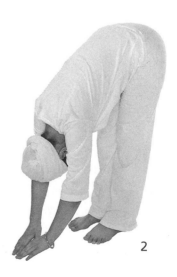

2. From this position, very slowly bend forward, keeping the arms straight and close to the ears. Stay down and inhale. Hold the breath as long as possible while pumping the Navel. Then exhale and pump the navel on the held exhale. Continue this process. **2 minutes**.

The above exercises prevent menopause and "Woman's Disease," characterized by insecurity and emotional behavior.

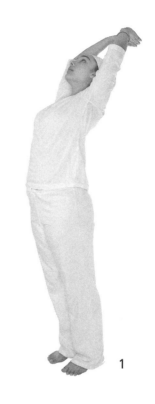

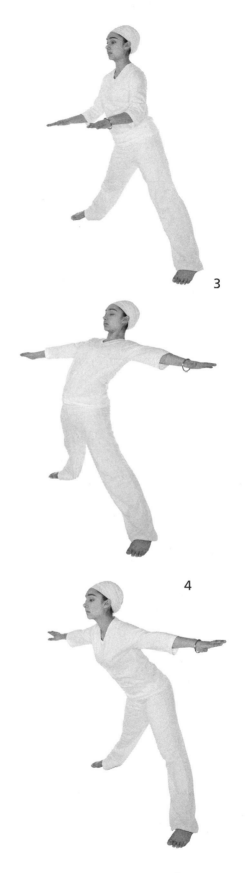

3. In a standing position, spread the legs as wide apart as possible without losing balance. Bend the elbows, and have the forearms more or less parallel to the ground. Begin rotating the hips at a moderate pace in as complete and large circles as possible. The direction can be either to the left or right. **2 minutes**.

This exercise hurts and works on an area that is never massaged and where you don't like to be hurt: the back of the spine. This exercise will raise the spirit, correct any victim mentality, and give the will to fight and not give in.

4. Maintain the same leg position as in Exercise 3, but straighten the arms. Begin a backward and alternate rotation of the arms, never bringing the arms more than 30 degrees in toward the body. The rhythm is one rotation of the arm per second. While rotating the arms, bend forward from the waist half way, straighten up again, and then bend backward from the waist. Rhythm: 15 seconds per complete cycle. **1 1/2 minutes**.

This exercise is for stamina, clear thinking and prevention of menopause.

5. **Deep Relaxation**. **10 minutes**.

A WOMAN'S MOON CENTERS

A woman is a highly sophisticated system. She must keep her energy systems finely tuned and balanced so she can honestly, intelligently, intuitively and consciously create every facet of life. There is a powerful relationship between woman and her lunar vibrations. This is manifested physically, mentally, & behaviorally. She waxes and wanes emotionally according to the movement of her "inner moon" relative to the influences of the outer Moon. The chin is the main center for receiving the moon's energies. This is true for both men and women. But while a man has just this one interaction with the moon, the woman has 11 additional centers through which the energy moves during a 28-day cycle. So at any one time, the chin and one of the other centers is activated, approximately 2 1/2 days each.

Listed below are the 11 Moon Centers and the emotional and behavioral changes that accompany that 2 1/2-day cycle.

One   ARCLINE. At the hairline. Most sensitive. Nothing can move her an inch. She is most authentic at this time.

Two   PINK OF THE CHEEKS. Lacking in restraint, and should watch her behavior carefully.

Three   LIPS. Rather than talking, she becomes extremely private.

Four   EARLOBES. Stimulates her to discuss values.

Five   BACK OF THE NECK. She wants to communicate at a very romantic frequency. Can be a bit foolish.

Six   BREASTS. Compassionate and giving.

Seven   NAVEL POINT. She is most insecure in this point of the cycle.

Eight   INNER THIGHS. She wants to confirm everything.

Nine   EYEBROWS. She is very imaginative and dreamy, building sand castles in the sky.

Ten/Eleven CLITORIS and INNER MEMBRANE OF VAGINA. She is very charming, eager to meet, talk, and socialize. External behaviors.

Once she starts to track these in herself and can recognize her own cycle, she can become much more conscious in her decision-making, actions, and relationships.

MEDITATION TO **BALANCE THE MOON CENTERS**

FEBRUARY 19, 1979

POSTURE: Lying on the stomach, place the chin on the ground, and keep the head straight. The arms are along side the body, with the palms of the hands facing up. *(This is a variation of Kirtan Kriya. See page 14 for more details.)*

EYES: Focused at the Brow Point.

MANTRA: The Panj Shabd: *SA TA NA MA*. Mentally vibrate the mantra in the following way:

SAA—Infinity, cosmos, beginning	*Press the Jupiter (index) finger and thumb.*
TAA—Life, existence	*Press the Saturn (middle) finger and thumb.*
NAA—Death, totality	*Press the Sun (ring) finger and thumb.*
MAA—Rebirth, resurrection	*Press the Mercury (pinkie) finger and thumb.*

The mantra chanted silently. Meditate on the sound current coming in through the crown of the head (the Tenth Gate) and flowing out through the center of the forehead (Third Eye Point), in an "L."

BREATH: The breath will regulate itself.

TIME: Continue for **3-31 minutes**.

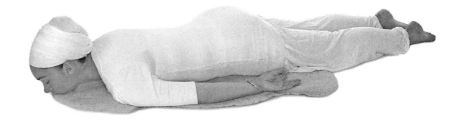

 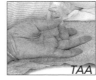 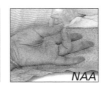 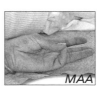

SAA   TAA   NAA   MAA

About This Meditation

This meditation is FOR WOMEN ONLY, and is the highest meditation for her. It is one of the most creative meditations, one can break any habit with it. This meditation balances the moon centers, the outer moon effect, the inner moon cycle, and one's own zodiac moon effect. It also balances the glandular system, and the movement between the 11 moon centers.

MEDITATION FOR DEEP RELAXATION

JULY 2, 1997

POSTURE: Sit in Easy Pose with a straight spine. If you are sitting on a chair, make sure the feet are flat on the ground, and the legs are not crossed. This is a requirement for this meditation.

MUDRA: Open the mouth and form an "O." Stick the tongue out of the right side of the mouth, to form a "Q." Keep the tongue out. If you have trouble holding the tongue in this position, hold it slightly between your teeth.
(Note: The tongue should NOT be straight out, but extended out to the right side of the mouth.)

BREATH: Breathe long and deep through the mouth, keeping the tongue extended throughout the meditation.

EYE FOCUS: Eyes are closed.

MANTRA: Any beautiful music can be played. *(Ardas Bhaee by Singh Kaur was played in the original class.)*

TIME: Done in class for **7 minutes**. If you ever need to deeply relax, try this on your own for **3 minutes**.

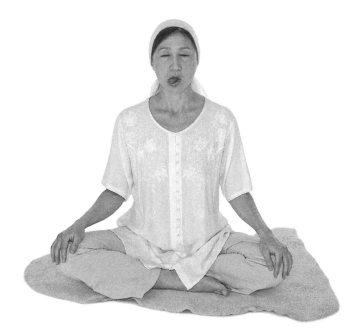

TO END: Hold the position, inhale and hold the breath **15 seconds**. Then squeeze the breath out with a powerful exhale through the mouth. Repeat, holding **10 seconds**. Then one last time, holding **5 seconds**. Relax.

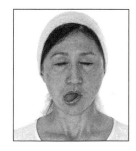

About This Meditation

There is no more powerful relaxation than this. When you are very nervous, and you have so many thoughts, and you are being ground up by everything, do this for **3 minutes**. You will be shocked—things will disappear. Karma will be over. It's called pre-experience. Your "Q" should be perfect.

FORTY STEPS TO BLISS
ANAND SAHIB OF GURU AMAR DAS
The Song of Bliss

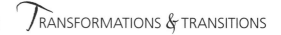

WISDOM COMES TO US AS A GIFT. We can only find it when humility brings us to the state of surrender. When we surrender, we become zero. And that zeroing out creates a vacuum for something new. As wisdom pours into the space created by the vacuum of surrender, we grow. We learn. And that learning transforms us, bringing the hope and the promise of a new and better day.

The *Anand Sahib* was birthed through such a profound moment of surrender. There are different versions of the story. Let me do the best I can to retell it here.

Guru Amar Das and the Old Yogi

One day a very old yogi came to visit the third teacher of the Sikhs, Guru Amar Das. Guru Amar Das had succeeded the second Sikh teacher, Guru Angad, in the year 1552. He lived in what is now northwestern India. By the time Guru Amar Das became the Guru, he was already an old man. He had lived life and he carried the unique perspective that comes with age into his reign as the Guru.

The yogi was also very old. He had spent years and years in isolation and deep meditation. The yogi had developed mastery over the elements, had acquired tremendous mystical powers—but still—there was something missing.

So the old yogi decided to visit the old Sikh Guru.

In audience with Guru Amar Das, and after paying the proper respects, the yogi described his frustration with his practice and then asked very simply, "Oh kind and wise Teacher, will you teach me how to just live life?"

Guru Amar Das nodded. "Leave this body," he told the yogi. "Be reborn in my family. Then come to me and I will teach you how to live."

The yogi took his leave of the Guru. And in obedience to the Guru's directive, sat down in meditation and left his body. In due time, the wife of Guru Amar Das's son Mohri gave birth to a grandson. When Guru Amar Das heard of the birth of the child, he knew that the yogi's soul had been reborn. Immediately he called for the child to be brought to him even though the traditional time of sequestering the infant with the mother had not yet passed. As soon as his grandson was brought before him, Guru Amar Das sang the *Anand Sahib*—the Song of Bliss. When he was done singing, the old Guru named the child Anand.

The Song of Bliss

What, then, is the *Anand Sahib*? It is a sacred teaching song in 40 verses, or steps, that give the essential lesson for the soul for the first 40 years of life. The first verse, or step, relates to the first year of life. The second verse, or step, to the second year. And so on until the age of 40. If each lesson is learned properly, and if grace is with the situation, then by the age of 40 one will have realized the experience of *Jiwan Mukht*, of being liberated while alive.

Yet even if the time of liberation has not yet come, the 40 steps of the *Anand Sahib* help to develop what the respected Sikh scholar Dr. Balkar Singh calls "the perfected human psyche." This is a psyche that has been thoroughly trained to support the reality of the soul in the midst of social and daily life. It is a mind whose senses can navigate the complexity of the human experience without losing touch with the Divine Spirit infused and prevailing through all. The perfected human psyche strives for the awareness

ਗੁਰੇੜ ਭਟਿਆ ਮੇਰੀ ਮਾਏ ਸਤਿਗੁਰੂ ਮੈ ਪਾਇਆ

of one's essential union with Divinity while living the daily duties of family life.

The thought is that with each year from birth until 40, a person is developing and maturing. At every stage of development, there is a unique lesson on how we anchor ourselves to our Spirit instead of being trapped in time and space. When a person learns these lessons, then bliss naturally happens. Bliss is that state where you are you, no matter what pressure you are under. When you can deliver your Self, your truth, your destiny in the face of every challenge and obstacle, then you know what bliss is. Then you are truly happy.

Ultimately, the perfected human psyche understands that spiritual development, like social development, is an organic process with a life of its own. We are each of us flowers in the Hands of a Master Gardener. And the time of our blooming depends on something greater than effort and intellect. This psyche moves with profound tolerance and love towards self and others, understanding the vastness of the Creative play and the uniqueness of the precious gift of human life.

Suggestions for Practice

You can meditate on the *Anand Sahib* in its entirety. Or you can focus on a single *pauri*, or verse, that relates to a specific year of your life—the year you are currently in, or a year where something happened that needs healing. Once you've chosen a *pauri* to work with, recite it 11 times a day, and see what happens. Use the *Anand Sahib* as a tool to further your yogic practice. And understand what Yogi Bhajan meant when he said, "Follow its words. Ask yourself questions. Befriend it. Practice it and live it. You will realize what you have with the *Anand Sahib*, and what Guru Amar Das gave you as the best gift."

EK ONG KAAR KAUR KHALSA
ESPAÑOLA, NEW MEXICO

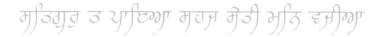

CROSSING OVER: A PRAN SUTRA

JULY 18, 1984

Shabd Guru

AT THE MOMENT OF DEATH, there will be a few seconds when you will be shown the panorama of your entire life. It is vital when we are confronted in those few seconds, that our mind connects with the majesty of the Undying Self, and the Reality of existence. Yogi Bhajan says this can be done with a *pran sutra*, a mantra that gives us this experience. When we can keep such a mantra in the mind during these three seconds, the connection with the Neutral Mind will be constant, and we will not react. We will not condemn ourselves, even when we "experience" the weaknesses or errors of our own life.

"By your own actions you may condemn yourself—that's a possibility. Normally, people do. Because you are going to see the waste of life that you've gone through, and say, "Oh my God, I did it again!" You follow? When you say, "I did it again," at that moment this one line may come to your memory:

ਪ੍ਰਭ ਜੀਉ ਖਸਮਾਨਾ ਕਰਿ ਪਿਆਰੇ
ਬੁਰੇ ਭਲੇ ਹਮ ਥਾਰੇ

Prabh jee-o khasmaanaa kar piaaray.
Buray bhalay ham thaaray.
Oh Beloved God, make me your own.
Good or bad, I am yours.
—Guru Arjan, Siri Guru Granth Sahib, page 631

"You can remember it in any other language, but naad is the only thing which can penetrate in that moment, through the death orbit. I am not here to push Gurmukhi on you, that is not my purpose. But I do want to push redemption on you—redempton at that moment. That moment is the moment of judgment, where you within you, stands and judges you.

"You may remember:

ਰਖੇ ਰਖਣਹਾਰਿ ਆਪਿ ਉਬਾਰਿਅਨੁ
ਗੁਰ ਕੀ ਪੈਰੀ ਪਾਇ ਕਾਜ ਸਵਾਰਿਅਨੁ

Rakhe rakhanhaar aap ubaariun.
Gur kee pairee paa-e kaaj savaariun
The Protector who shields all has liberated me.
By falling at the feet of the Guru my life
was made beautiful.
—Guru Arjan, Siri Guru Granth Sahib, page 517

"Or, you may just remember the middle of a shabd, any shabd. If any one line of 1430 pages can come in, that's all that is needed—just one line.

Let me give you an experiment. If tomorrow a problem comes, just remember who your teacher is. Just remember at that time who your teacher is. You will find a solution. And if that solution really comes through to you, then believe it—and then, remember some portion of the Siri Guru Granth Sahib; so that on that final day, all you have to remember at that time is just one line, one sutra.

"Here's another example:

ਅਨੰਦੁ ਭਇਆ ਮੇਰੀ ਮਾਏ ਸਤਿਗੁਰੂ ਮੈ ਪਾਇਆ

Anand bhaiaa mere maae, satiguroo mai paaiaa.
Oh my Mother I am in Ecstasy.
I am truly in Ecstasy! For I have realized my True Guru.
—Guru Amar Das, Siri Guru Granth Sahib, page 917

"This is the first sutra of the Anand Sahib. Do you want to know what this can do? If you are dying from a disease, and your body is so rotten that doctors have given up, use this one line. You can be healed; it delivers miracles."

Suggestions for Practice

Yogi Bhajan said that every individual has their own *pran sutra*—that line or two from the morning's *Japji Sahib*, or a single verse from a *shabd* that won't let go. Find your own *pran sutra* by listening, deeply listening.

There are however, master keys, such as the ones suggested above. The master key, or *pran sutra*, that Yogi Bhajan suggested we practice throughout the day, every day, so when that final day comes, we have it written on our hearts, were these lines from *Dhan Dhan Ram Das Gur*:

ਨਾਨਕੁ ਤੂ ਲਹਣਾ ਤੂਹੈ
ਗੁਰੁ ਅਮਰੁ ਤੂ ਵੀਚਾਰਿਆ
ਗੁਰੁ ਡਿਠਾ ਤਾਂ ਮਨੁ ਸਾਧਾਰਿਆ

ਧੰਨੁ ਧੰਨੁ ਰਾਮਦਾਸ ਗੁਰੁ
ਜਿਨਿ ਸਿਰਿਆ ਤਿਨੈ ਸਵਾਰਿਆ

Nanak too(n) lehna too(n) hai,
Guru amar too(n) veecharia
Guru ditta tan man sadaria

Dhan dhan ram das gur,
jinae siria tinae sevaria

You are Nanak, you are Angad,
And Guru Amar Das; I recognize this in you
Seeing the Guru, my soul is comforted!

Praise, Praise Guru Ram Das!
The Creator has adorned & embellished you!
—Siri Guru Granth Sahib, page 968

ਧੰਨੁ ਧੰਨੁ ਰਾਮਦਾਸ ਗੁਰੁ ਜਿਨਿ ਸਿਰਿਆ ਤਿਨੈ ਸਵਾਰਿਆ

HEALING & RELAXATION

BECOMING HEALTHY, HAPPY & HOLY

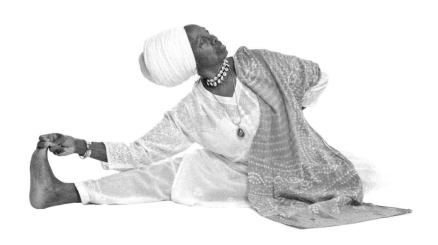

I AM A WOMAN is a very relaxed state of mind, a place where our intuition can guide us. Do you know how much time that can save, if we only trusted it? In seven seconds we can know the answer.

IN TODAY'S WORLD, EVERY WOMAN I KNOW, no matter what their age—from teenager to octogenarian—is busy, and in the busyness of our business, we often forget ourselves. We put our work and the needs of others in the forefront, which in the short-term may work out fine; but in the long-run, it leads to deficiency and burnout. We will never get everything done—that is a fact. So with that as our premise, how do we make choices that serve others—and ourselves?

Our true impact comes from a relaxed state of being, the state where we can connect to the Infinite within us and within every other being on the planet. "I Am a Woman," is a very relaxed state of mind, a place where our intuition can guide us. Do you know how much time that can save, if we only trusted it? In seven seconds we can know the answer, which otherwise could take days of analysis, comparisons, charts and discussions.

To relax, we must move and meditate. **The Movement Relaxation Kriya** in this chapter releases the imprint of emotions and traumas on our bodies and our minds. This powerful technology allows us to experience our Self and our identity as a woman. When we see ourselves as the True Self, and value this state, we can automatically bless ourselves and others. To heal others we must heal ourselves first. Through our power to bless and heal, beyond time and space, we can heal the planet. Yogi Bhajan was very clear: "How can you bless someone else if you cannot bless yourself?" The meditation, **Bless Yourself**, is a powerful technology to practice this self-blessing, first thing in the morning and throughout the day.

In this relaxed state of being rather than state of doing, all women are healers. All women—you, me, the 1-year-old child and the 16-year-old teenager—have always been healers. Without this art we would not have survived on the planet. Through the practice of the **Ra Ma Da Sa Meditation** we can send this powerful prayer and blessing across time and space. Yogi Bhajan told us that by practicing this meditation our touch and our look will heal.

"I am a woman, I am relaxed, I bless and heal myself and others through my presence and my prayer."

What a powerful self-affirmation this is. Enjoy your practice of this technology as we heal ourselves and heal the planet in the Aquarian Age.

HARI CHARN KAUR KHALSA
ESPAÑOLA, NEW MEXICO

GETTING THE BODY OUT OF DISTRESS

AUGUST 22, 1986

1. Sit with the legs straight out in front. Using both hands alternately, begin slapping the tops of the thighs. **30 seconds**.

The point you are stimulating is where the Third Meridian, liver, and kidney meet.

2. Keeping the legs stretched out straight, cup the kneecaps with each hand. Massage each kneecap with a circular motion. Massage with force and motion. **2 minutes**.

Underneath the kneecap regulates and sustains your body's water. Too much water in your system can create headaches; too little water can create bitchiness and itchiness without reason. Your knee has an important effect on your well-being. The majority of us walk incorrectly and the knees take tremendous stress.

3. Locate the point one-hand-width *below* the knee, on the outside of each calf, right below where the fibula bone protrudes. Vigorously pound the muscle at that point on each side. **2 minutes**.

This is a general energy point in acupuncture. Stimulating it can totally change your metabolism. Pound harder and heavier for the second minute.

4. Repeat Exercise 2, massaging the knees for **10 seconds**.

5. Locate the point one-hand-width *above* the knee on the inside of the thigh. Make fists of your hands and alternately pound the muscle at that point on each side. **1 minute**.

This is a sex point. It may hurt in some cases. It will let you know that there is something happening in your

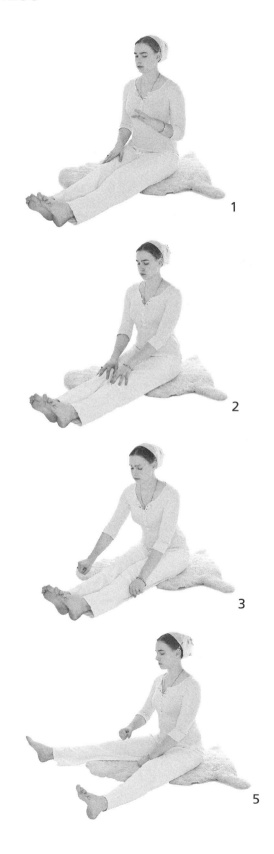

spine, in your shoulders, and in your head.

6. Spread the legs wide apart, grab the outside of the ankles, firmly holding the Achilles tendons. Move the torso up and down between the legs, keeping the knees straight. Move fast. **1 1/2 minutes**. (An alternate position for this exercise is sitting in Full Lotus holding onto the big toes.) Move fast like a propeller that moves so fast nobody can see the blades.

This balances the flow of energy in the spine. Move with a rhythm as fast as you can.

7. Sit in Easy Pose. Form the hands into a tepee, touching fingertips to fingertips at the Heart Center. Rotate the joined fingertips together, moving the fingertips in a circular motion while the wrists stay steady. **1 minute**.

The previous exercise will have little benefit unless you do this exercise after it. It sends the energy equally to 72,000 nerve channels. Kundalini energy, the spiral force, the diagonal force, can be moved to every part of the body just by this movement, providing you have correctly stimulated the energy to begin with.

8. Lie down on the back with the arms on the floor beside the body, palms down. Begin rapidly raising and lowering the hips. This motion will bounce the hips against the ground, giving them a vigorous massage. Create a sound like galloping horses. Move fast, have a beautiful intercourse with God. **2 minutes**.

9. Still lying on the back, make the hands into fists. Bend the elbows and hit the shoulders with the fists. Then raise the arms straight up to 90 degrees. Keep the arms straight and lower them back down to the sides, hitting the ground hard with open palms. Make the hands back into fists once again, hit the shoulders, and continue the sequence. **1 minute**.

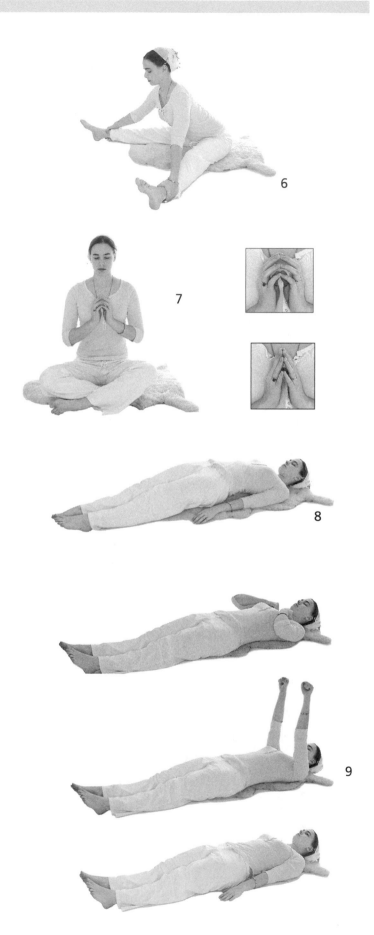

10. Still on the back alternately hit the chest with open palms. **1 minute**.

11. Still on the back, alternately tap the forehead with open palms. **30 seconds**.

12. Still on the back, grasp the heels. Roll back and forth on the spine. Roll along the whole spine, from hips to neck. **1 minute**.

This will equalize the energy in the spine and will comfort your lower triangle.

13. Still on your back, move like a snake. The hips move in one direction while shoulders and rib cage move in the other direction. Start out just moving one-hundredth of a millimeter in each direction. This is a very small and precise movement. **2 minutes**. *Move with small movements, but with force—bottom to top. Give the spinal energy its own chance to move and give the vertebrae an adjustment.*

14. Lie down flat and relax. Breathe slowly and deeply at the Navel Point. **1 1/2 minutes**.

15. **Cat Stretch** slowly left and right. **I minute**.

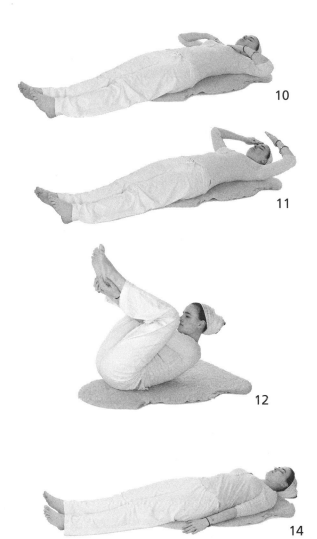

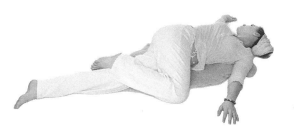

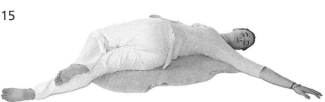

15

16. Lie flat on the back, pull the chin in and raise the head and neck up. Leave the shoulders relaxed on the ground, hands flat on the ground at your sides. Your body is relaxed, but your neck is lifted and tense. **1 minute**.

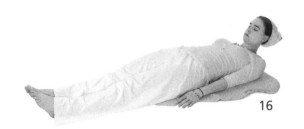

17. Relax, close your eyes for **2 minutes**. Then come sitting up in Easy Pose and assess your body's energy.

TO END: This kriya ends with a brief self-massage:

Using your thumbs, massage under your cheek bones. **15 seconds**.

Use the base of your palms to massage your jaw area in a circular motion. **20 seconds**.

Use the first three fingers of each hand to massage the sides of the neck. **10 seconds**.

Place your palms over your ears and massage your ears in a circular motion. **30 seconds**.

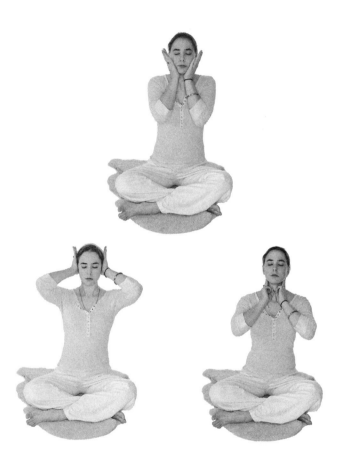

About This Kriya

This moves the energy in every part of the body systematically. This kriya can bring great change. It is a good set of exercises to do every day, because if the body's energy is not released, circulated, and distributed, then it will start malfunctioning.

"When the finite gets to you and you show your Infinity—that is Divinity"

— Yogi Bhajan

MOVEMENT RELAXATION SERIES

AUGUST 22, 1986

1. Stand straight with arms completely relaxed. Close the eyes. Feel any tension in each part of the body and consciously let it go. Next, begin to sway and move every part of the body. Dance gracefully feeling the easy movement of each body area. If there is gentle rhythmic music of a high vibration available, it may be used as a background. Continue for **3 to 11 minutes**. The time can be extended as long as you enjoy it.

2. Immediately stand straight with the eyes still closed. With the hands, begin to lightly feel each part and area of the body without reservation. Every square inch must be touched. Feel sensitivity with the palms. Continue for **3 to 5 minutes**.

3. Lean forward with arms hanging completely relaxed. All the muscles of the body should be relaxed. Let the breath be normal.
Continue for **3 to 11 minutes**.

4. Inhale and exhale deeply several times. Then, slowly lean backwards with arms hanging loosely down. Breath is relaxed. Hold for **1 minute**. Then completely relax on your back for **10 minutes**.

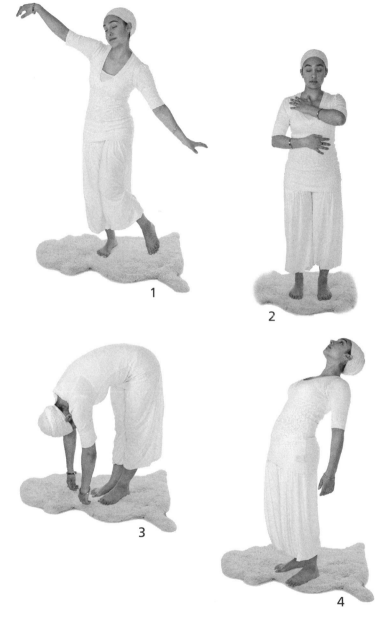

About This Kriya

This is a very beautiful movement meditation kriya which will relax your whole body and mind. It is important for every woman to deeply relax on a daily basis. Stress which builds up can cause physical and mental imbalances and this short yoga set is a beautiful way to release tension in the mind and body.

Rhythmic, unforced, graceful, and free movement relaxes the entire body and releases the tensions we store in the body from our daily emotions. All emotional traumas leave their signature of tension in the body, which need to be released. Feeling the entire body confirms the reality of the relaxation and smoothes the aura.

The other exercises strengthen the heart and circulatory system. If this system is weak, then tissues will tense and the joints will build up deposits that create illness, making true, deep relaxation difficult. This simple series is for total relaxation and a cooperative coordination of mind and body into the experience of Self.

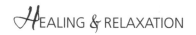

MEDITATION TO **RELAX AND REJOICE**

FEBRUARY 19, 1979

POSTURE: Sit in Easy Pose with a straight spine. Be relaxed in this position.

MUDRA: Make a fist of the left hand with the thumb inside. Wrap the right hand around the left fist, placing the right thumb over the base of the left thumb. The elbows are relaxed down by the sides.

EYE FOCUS: Focus on the tip of the nose.

BREATH: Inhale deeply. Chant the following mantra in a monotone:

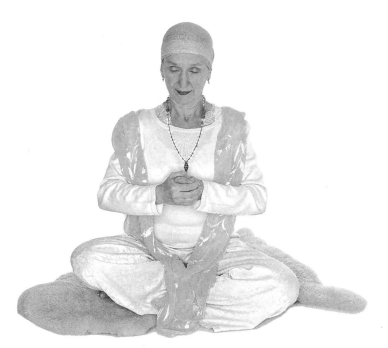

HAREE HAR HAREE HAR
HAREE HAR HAREE HAR
HAREE HAR HAREE HAR
HAREE HAR HAREE HAR

TIME: Begin by practicing for **11 minutes**. You may gradually build up to 62 minutes and even 2-1/2 hours.

About This Meditation

This meditation is to help you relax and rejoice. It enables you to understand the contrast between working from your ego and working from your inner self, from your soul, aligned with the Will of God. Allow yourself free time to ground yourself after doing this meditation.

PADMANI KRIYA: ENERGIZING AND HEALING
AUGUST 12, 1977

POSTURE: Sit in Easy Pose with the spine straight.

MUDRA: Bring the elbows together in front of the chest, forearms touching from the elbows to the wrists. Make a lotus of the hands by stretching the fingers out straight and apart from one another. Allow the Mercury (pinkie) fingers to touch at the tips; the thumbs touch along the sides of the first joint and are stretched toward the chest.

EYE FOCUS: Focus the eyes to look through the triangle formed by the little fingers.

BREATH: Inhale slowly and deeply through the nose until the lungs are completely full. Then close off both nostrils by placing the tips of the joined thumbs against these openings. After retaining the breath as long as possible, move the thumbs slightly away from the nostrils again and hold the breath out as long as possible. Inhale and continue.

MANTRA: One can mentally focus on any mantra.

TIME: Begin with **3 minutes** and gradually increase to **11 minutes**.

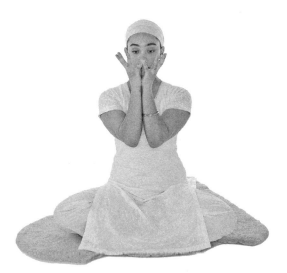

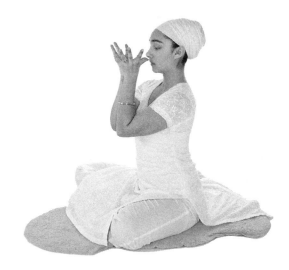

About This Meditation

This kriya is FOR WOMEN ONLY. It is the most beautiful way to do *pranayam*. It is simple and generates a lot of energy. If there is any area of the body that needs to be strengthened, mentally concentrate on that area while practicing this *pranayam*.

MEDITATION TO **COMPLETELY NEUTRALIZE TENSION**
SEPTEMBER 29, 1977

POSTURE: Sit in Easy Pose with a straight spine, and a light Neck Lock.

MUDRA: With both palms facing up at the Heart Center, cross the right palm over the left palm. Place the left thumb in the center of the right palm and cross the right thumb over the left thumb.

EYE FOCUS: The eyes are 9/10 closed. As the meditation progresses, they may close all the way.

BREATH & MANTRA: Deeply inhale and chant Long Sat Nam's in a ratio of 35 to 1. You may begin with a ratio of 12 to 1 and build up to the longer practice.

> *SAAAAAAAAT NAAM*

TIME: Begin with **11 minutes** and build up to **31 minutes**.

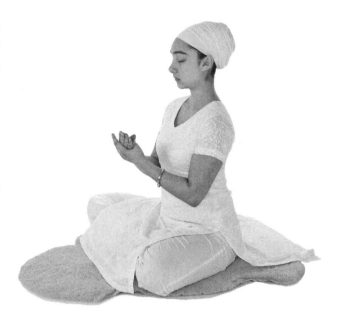

About This Meditation

This is an extremely relaxing meditation. It completely neutralizes tension, and puts you in a most relaxed state. By doing the meditation for 40 days, you can revitalize your glandular system and reestablish glandular equilibrium.

MEDITATION TO **BLESS YOURSELF**

APRIL 19, 2000

POSTURE: Sit in Easy Pose with a straight spine, and a light Neck Lock.

MUDRA: Raise both arms out to the sides, bend the elbows so that the forearms come to a 90 degree angle, fingers pointing to the sky. Hands face forward.

EYE FOCUS: Eyes are focused at the tip of the nose.

MANTRA & MOVEMENT: Chant along with Nirinjan Kaur's recording of *Humee Hum Brahm Hum*, and move in rhythm with the mantra:

HUMEE HUM

Touch the top of your head with the left hand, blessing yourself.

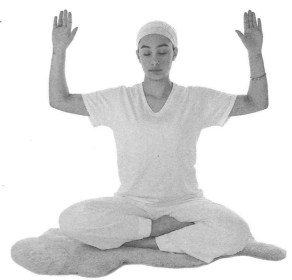

BRAHM HUM

Return to the starting position.

TIME: Continue for **11 minutes**.

TO END: Inhale, hold the breath, tighten the spine, and stiffen the left hand. Pull the energy of the spine into the left hand. Exhale. Repeat 2 more times. Relax.

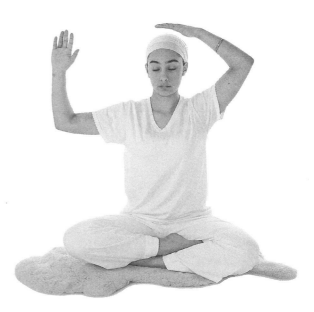

About This Meditation

When you get up in the morning, stretch yourself with cat stretch. Then lie down straight with your right arm alongside you, and bless yourself as you did in the meditation. One blessing is enough to start your day. Start living consciously. Become a human being. Be humble, serviceful, kind, compassionate. Your power to heal is in how much anger you have forgiven yourself for.

RA MA DA SA HEALING MEDITATION

POSTURE: Sit in an Easy Pose with a straight spine, and a light Neck Lock.

MUDRA: Have the elbows tucked comfortably against the ribs. Extend the forearms out at a 45-degree angle out from the center of the body. The palms are flat, facing up, the wrists pulled back, fingers together. Consciously keep the palms flat during the meditation.

MANTRA: The Siri Gaitri mantra, which consists of eight basic sounds: *RA MA DA SA SA SAY SO HUNG* and is sung in following way:

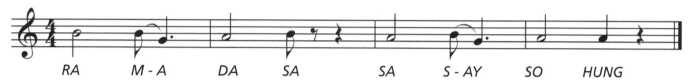

Pull in the Navel Point powerfully on the sound *HUNG*. Forcefully clip off the sound *HUNG* as you pull in the navel. Chant one complete cycle of the mantra. Then inhale deeply and repeat. Move the mouth fully with each sound. Feel the resonance in the mouth and the sinus areas. Let your mind concentrate on the qualities that are evoked by the combination of sounds.

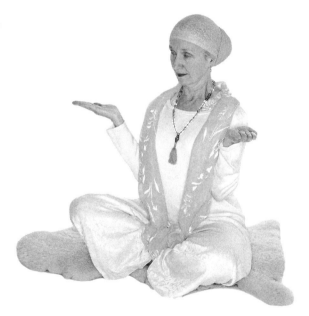

TIME: Chant powerfully for **11-31 minutes**.

TO END: Inhale deeply and hold the breath as you offer a healing prayer, visualizing the person you wish to heal (including yourself) as being healthy, radiant, and strong. Imagine the person completely engulfed in healing white light, completely healed. Then exhale and inhale deeply again, hold the breath and offer your prayer. Then, lift your arms up high and vigorously shake out your hands and fingers.

About This Meditation

Certain mantras are to be cherished like a beautiful gem. The Siri Gaitri Mantra is just such a jewel. It is unique, and it captures the radiant healing energy of the Cosmos as a gem captures the light of the Sun. Like a gem it can be put into many settings for different purposes and occasions. When Yogi Bhajan first shared this technology he gave a series of meditations that use the inner dynamics of this mantra. If you master any of these practices you will be rewarded with healing and awareness.

The mantra is also a Sushmuna Mantra. It has eight sounds that stimulate the kundalini to flow in the central channel of the spine and in the chakras, accompanied by metabolic adjustment to the new level of energy in the body, and balances the five zones of the left and right hemispheres of the brain to activate the Neutral Mind.

The mantra uses a sound current. The sounds create a juxtaposition of energies.

RAA is the energy of the Sun: strong, bright, and hot. It energizes and purifies.

MAA is the energy of the Moon: receptive, cool, and nurturing.

DAA is the energy of Earth: secure and personal. It is the ground of action.

SAA is the impersonal Infinity. The cosmos in all of its dimensions openness and expansivness and totality is *SAA*.

Then the mantra repeats the sound; this repetition is a turning point. The first part of the mantra is ascending and expands into the Infinite. The second part of the mantra pivots those qualities of the highest and most subtle ether, and brings them back down. It interweaves the ether with the earth.

SAA is the impersonal Infinity.

SAY is the totality of experience and is personal. It is the feeling of a sacred "Thou." It is the embodiment of *SAA*.

SO is the personal sense of merger and Identity.

HUNG is the Infinite, vibrating and real. The two qualities together (*SO* and *HUNG*) mean: *"I am Thou."*

As you chant this mantra you complete a cycle of energy and go through a circuit of the chakras. You grow toward the Infinite, then you convert the link between the finite and Infinite at *SAA*. Then you revert back to an embodiment of purity.

HEALING THROUGH IDENTITY
Jap Man Sat Nam

Shabd Guru

REPEAT, O MY MIND, the truth of my identity—Sat Nam, Sat Nam. These words are the essence of this *shabd*, which is said to bring deep relaxation and healing to the Self. Most of our anxiety and stress comes from resistance—resistance to what is. We find ourselves constantly trying to control, manage, persuade, manipulate—whatever word you want to use—our surroundings, our relationships, our environments and even our own identity, in order to make everything okay. Part of this resistance to what is comes from our childhood—the 'good girl' complex—where we tried to be what our parents wanted us to be; and part of our resistance comes from cultural conditioning, which demands that we look right, act right, 'be' right—a projection of the same childhood fears and insecurities. What if, instead, we relaxed into the true nature of our identity—Sat Nam? Feel your Navel Point relax, just by posing this question.

This *shabd* reminds us that prosperity and peace come as the natural result, the fruit of that *bij*, or seed, Sat Nam. Seeing your identity as true, beyond any role you may play, any responsibilities or check lists, and relaxing into that true identity brings great healing. When you merge with that identity through meditation, the repetition of the Name—you become radiant and disaster runs away from you. Why? Because you're in the flow of the creativity of your identity: You expand rather than contract. You accept rather than push away. You breathe in and you breathe out. You're in balance with all that is. In this way you cross the world ocean of maya and merge into your truth—one with God—which is the deepest healing that can be obtained.

Suggestions for Practice

Play this *shabd* while you sleep or sing it before going to bed. In this way your mind is elevated through the Gurbani, and your soul begins to vibrate with the reality of Sat Nam. Consciously release all other identities and roles: wife, mother, daughter, professional, friend, even woman, and merge into the single identity of Sat Nam. Breathe deeply in that space and know that all peace and prosperity come to you through this sound current.

SAT PURKH KAUR KHALSA
ESPAÑOLA, NEW MEXICO

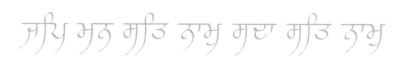

ਜਾਪਿ ਮਨ ਸਤਿ ਨਾਮੁ ਸਦਾ ਸਤਿ ਨਾਮੁ

HEALING THROUGH IDENTITY
JAP MAN SAT NAM
Guru Ram Das, Siri Guru Granth Sahib, page 669

ਧਨਾਸਰੀ ਮਹਲਾ 4
ਇਛਾ ਪੂਰਕੁ ਸਰਬ ਸੁਖਦਾਤਾ ਹਰਿ ਜਾ ਕੈ ਵਸਿ ਹੈ ਕਾਮਧੇਨਾ
ਸੋ ਐਸਾ ਹਰਿ ਧਿਆਈਐ ਮੇਰੇ ਜੀਅੜੇ
ਤਾ ਸਰਬ ਸੁਖ ਪਾਵਹਿ ਮੇਰੇ ਮਨਾ ॥1॥
ਜਪਿ ਮਨ ਸਤਿ ਨਾਮੁ ਸਦਾ ਸਤਿ ਨਾਮੁ
ਹਲਤਿ ਪਲਤਿ ਮੁਖ ਊਜਲ ਹੋਈ ਹੈ
ਨਿਤ ਧਿਆਈਐ ਹਰਿ ਪੁਰਖੁ ਨਿਰੰਜਨਾ ॥ ਰਹਾਉ ॥
ਜਹ ਹਰਿ ਸਿਮਰਨ ਭਇਆ ਤਹ ਉਪਾਧਿ ਗਤੁ ਕੀਨੀ
ਵਡਭਾਗੀ ਹਰਿ ਜਪਨਾ
ਜਨ ਨਾਨਕ ਕਉ ਗੁਰਿ ਇਹ ਮਤਿ ਦੀਨੀ ਜਪਿ ਹਰਿ ਭਵਜਲ ਤਰਨਾ ॥2॥6॥12॥

DHANAASAREE Mahelaa Chautha
Ichaa poorak sarb sukhdaataa har jaa kai vas hai kaamdhaynaa
So aisaa har dhiaa-ee-ai mayray jeearay
Taa sarb sukh paaveh mayray manaa.
Jap man sat nam sadaa sat naam
Halat palat mukh oojal hocc hai
Nit dhiaa-ee-ai har purakh niranjanaa (Rahao)
Jeh har simran bhaiaa te upaadh gat keenee
Vadhbhaagee har japnaa
Jan naanak kau gur eh mat deenee Jap har bhavjal tarnaa 2/6/12

RAAG DHANAASAREE, FOURTH CHANNEL OF LIGHT
The Lord is the Fulfiller of desires, the Giver of total peace; the Kaamadhaynaa, the wish-fulfilling cow, is in His power.
So meditate on such a Lord, O my soul. Then, you shall obtain total peace, O my mind. ‖ 1 ‖
Chant, O my mind, the True Name, Sat Naam, the True Name.
In this world, and in the world beyond, your face shall be radiant,
by meditating continually on the immaculate Lord God. ‖ Pause ‖
Wherever anyone remembers the Lord in meditation, disaster runs away from that place.
By great good fortune, we meditate on the Lord.
The Guru has blessed servant Nanak with this understanding,
that by meditating on the Lord, we cross over the terrifying world ocean. ‖ 2 ‖ 6 ‖ 12 ‖

BEAUTY BEGINS WITHIN

*Personal Discipline &
the Graceful Woman*

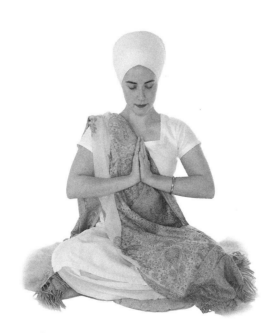

A WOMAN'S BEAUTY COMES FROM WITHIN—no amount of makeup can create that inner light. Her radiance, her inner light, is the fruit of those seeds of discipline, which she plants each day, in ways both large and small. Her body, when in balance, serves to expand that light to all—out of balance is another story—which is why in the 3HO way of life, healthy comes first for a reason. A healthy body is the foundation for a happy life. Anyone who's ever been ill, from the common cold to a chronic illness, knows how profoundly your health affects your ability to stabilize mood, emotion, and the will to act. A woman's body is her temple. In order to fulfill her highest potential and serve with grace, efficacy and integrity, a woman's body must be able to stand the test of time. Resilience and vitality are virtues of the disciplined, graceful woman.

Every woman has her own karmas, and the body often plays a role in expressing those karmas; illness and aging will come. But health and vitality are also available and can be cultivated. The practices described in the companion volume, *I AM A WOMAN: Creative, Sacred & Invincible*, go a long way toward establishing habits that promote health and vitality: cold shower therapy, self-massage, healing foods and nutrition, and even skin and hair care elevate a woman's consciousness, cleanse her endocrine system and support a strong sympathetic-parasympathetic response in the nervous system.

In addition to these simple disciplines, we have selected five basic kriyas that support the fundamental systems of a woman's health, radiance and long-term vitality. A woman's elimination system, the skin, lymph and bowel, are crucial to long-term health. These three kriyas address these fundamental organ systems, stimulating the regular excretion of waste and toxins, purifying the blood, and boosting a woman's radiance—inside and out.

A woman's flexibility, especially in the spine, is also vital for maintaining long-term youth and health. The kriya, **Self-Adjustment of the Spine**, naturally adjusts the sacrum and the pelvis in relation to the lower spine. Stability and flexibility in the pelvis affects a woman's entire cranio-sacral pulse, which when regular and smooth contributes to overall health and efficiency in the nervous system.

Finally, we've included the classic, simple set, **The Four U's**, which tonifies the entire body, strengthening, relaxing and healing the spine, inner organs, and the heart.

The glands are the guardians of a woman's health. Each of these kriyas address the endocrine system in their own unique way. The health of the glandular system is essential in maintaining a healthy and balanced hormonal response. When the hormones are out of balance, they can adversely affect a woman's emotional well-being, her ability to maintain a healthy weight, and can contribute to lethargy and chronic fatigue. In balance, a woman's hormones are her gift and the key to her youth and vitality.

These kriyas are the body's regular maintenance schedule. Just as you would never let your car go without gas, or a change of oil, don't allow your body to go without one of these kriyas for too long. They will help you maintain your youth, vitality and flexibility so that you're better able to "obey, serve, love and excel" and fulfill the essence of these teachings.

SAT PURKH KAUR KHALSA
ESPAÑOLA, NEW MEXICO

HEALTHY BOWEL SYSTEM

JULY 4, 1977

1. Stand with feet slighly wider than shoulder width apart. Bring the arms straight out to the sides, parallel to the ground. Palms are down. Bend forward from the waist, twist toward the left, bringing the right hand to the left foot and the left arm straight up.
Rhythm: About 10 seconds per cycle. Then switch to the opposite foot and hand.
TIME: 1 minute on each side.

Continue the same motion but alternating sides, and hold the hand on the foot for 5 seconds.
TIME: 3 minutes.

Continue the same alternating motion, and hold the hand on the foot for 25 seconds.
TIME: 2 minutes.

Finally, hold the position for **2 minutes** on each side.

RELAX: 2-3 minutes.

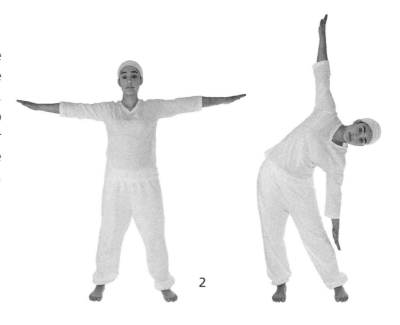

2. With legs still wide apart, arms parallel to the floor and palms down, bend to the side from the waist, letting the left arm come down the left side, and letting the right arm come straight up. Keep the spine in a single plane; don't allow the shoulder girdle to twist forward or back. Come back to the original position. Then stretch down the right side, and return to the original position.
Rhythm: **5 seconds** per side.
TIME: 1 minute.

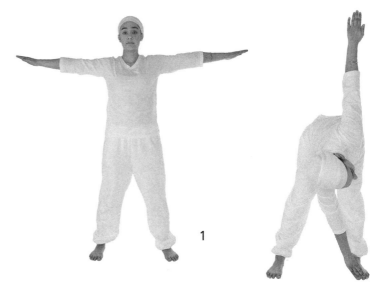

3. Begin in the same position as the previous exercise. Twist the torso and arms all the way to the left, then back to the original position. Then twist around to the right side, and finally back to the center. Keep the arms in a straight line with each other.
Rhythm: **2-3 seconds** per complete cycle.
TIME: 1 minute.

4. **Deep Relaxation**. Relax for **10 minutes**.

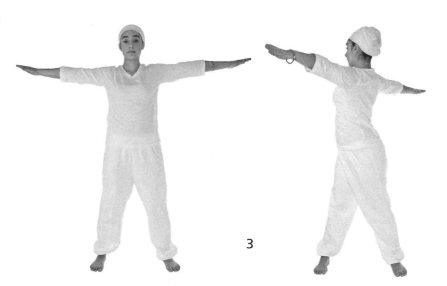

3

About This Kriya

This kriya works on the bowel system, and the First Chakra, important for good health. Normally when a woman is becoming sick, her bowel movements serve as an early indicator. It is suggested to do these exercises for 30 minutes a day for good health.

KRIYA TO MAKE YOUR SKIN RADIANT

FEBRUARY 26, 1986

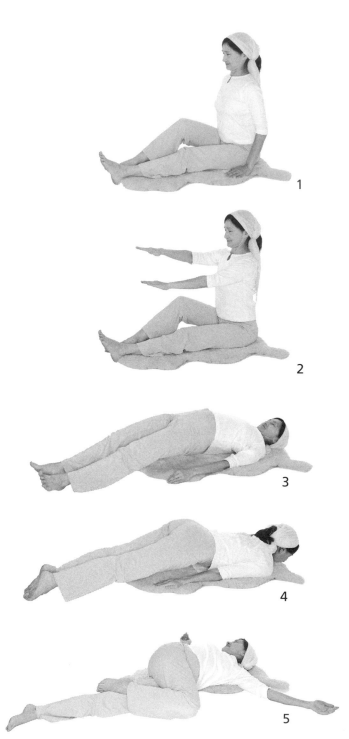

1. Sit with the legs stretched out in front, arms at the sides. Keeping the heels on the ground, bend and raise the left knee. As you lower the left knee, bend and raise the right knee, so that you alternately move the knees up and down. **3 minutes.**

2. Continue the same leg motion as in Exercise 1. Stretch the arms straight out in front, palms facing down. Begin alternately moving the arms up and down, coordinating with the leg motion, so that the left knee and arm move together, and the right knee and arm move together. Move at a speed of 5 times per second, or faster, and try to create a sweat. **15 minutes.**

3. Lie on the back with the arms at the sides. Raise and lower the pelvis so that everything from the shoulders to the ankles is lifted off the ground, then lowered back down. Move very quickly. **9 minutes.**

4. Same exercise as #3, but instead of lying on the back, lie on the stomach. **13 minutes.**

5. **Cat Stretch** alternately to the left side, then to the right side. Do as many as you can. **4 minutes.**

6. **Deep relaxation.** Lie down and relax. Breathe extremely slowly. **11 minutes.**

About This Kriya

Stress and anger affect the skin. Inner anger can make you accomplish a lot, but if you are angry and blaming, then this anger will keep you in a state of low self-esteem. This creates long-term stress which dulls the mind, makes life boring, and takes away your happiness. This set of exercises works to improve the skin by removing the effects of long-term anger and stress through adjustment of the metabolism.

KRIYA FOR THE LYMPH GLANDS
GLANDS ARE THE GUARDIANS OF HEALTH

OCTOBER 26, 1983

1. Sit in Easy Pose. Place the fingers on top of the head, the thumbs completely closing off the ears. In this position, begin twisting from side to side, keeping each motion separate. Move left, center, right, center, and so on. Keep the elbows up. **3 minutes**.

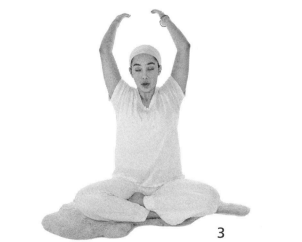

2. Still in Easy Pose, press the thumbs on the Mercury Mounds (just beneath the pinkie fingers). Bend the elbows and hold the hands near the shoulders, palms toward you. Pull Neck Lock, with chin in and chest out throughout the exercise. Begin raising alternate arms up high to a 60 degree angle, keeping the palms facing in. One hand goes up as the other goes down, in a push-pull motion. Move powerfully. The breath will become like a powerful Breath of Fire. Try to tire yourself out doing this. **3-4 minutes**.

This exercise stimulates the lymph glands of the arms and chest.

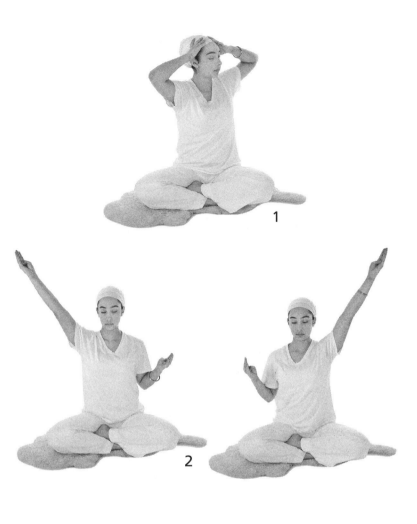

3. Still in Easy Pose, place the hands on the knees, palms facing up. The hands are relaxed but firm. Inhale through the mouth as you lift the arms high up and way back over the head, as if lifting something very powerfully. On the inhale, make a deep sound of heavy breathing with the mouth open wide, lips rounded in an "O." As the exercise continues, this sound will become like a lion's roar. As you exhale through the mouth, return the hands to the knees. Move powerfully. **4-5 minutes**.

It is all right if the hands don't land on the knees. It is more important for the arms to go way back over the head. The elbows may bend a little as the arms go up.

4. Still sitting, press the thumbs on the mounds beneath the Mercury (little) fingers, and close the fingers over the thumbs to make solid fists. Extend the arms straight out to the sides, palm-side of fists facing down. Moving quickly, lower the fists about a foot, the return them to the horizontal. Repeat the movement. Then quickly raise the arms up overhead and back to the horizontal. Repeat the motion. Keep the movements separate and rhythmical. Continue the 4-part sequence—down, down, up, up—for **3 minutes**.

Done powerfully, the motions become automatic. The breath will carry you through. You will breathe through every pore of the body. The sympathetic and parasympathetic nervous systems will come into balance. If you have drunk a lot of coffee in your life, you may find this exercise difficult to do.

5. Squat down in **Frog Pose**, on the toes, knees wide apart. Heels are touching, and raised up off the ground. Place the fingertips on the ground between the knees. The face is forward. Inhale as you raise the hips up, keeping the fingertips on the ground, heels up, knees locked. Exhale down, face forward, knees outside of arms. Continue rapidly for **3-4 minutes**.

6. Lie down on the back. Place the hands in Venus Lock under the neck. Bring the legs up and begin a bicycling motion, as if you were riding a bicycle in the air. The movement is not the piston push-pull, but rather the feet move in big circles. **3 minutes**.

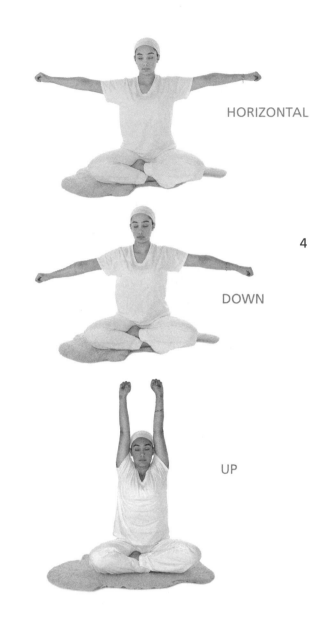

HORIZONTAL

4

DOWN

UP

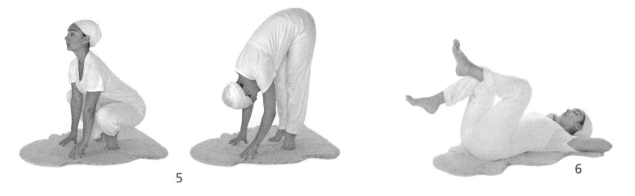

5

6

7. **Shoulder Stand**. From lying on the back, place the hands on the hips, just below the waist, and bring the hips and legs up to a vertical position, spine and legs perpendicular to the ground. Support the weight of the body on the elbows and shoulders using the hands to support the lower spine. The chin is pressed into the chest. Begin a bicycling motion. **2-3 minutes**.

8. Bring the legs back down over the head into **Plow Pose**. Alternate touching the toes to the ground in a scissor motion. Move quickly and powerfully. Keep up for 1 minutes.
This exercise helps prevent backaches.

9. Sit up in Easy Pose. Stretch the spine straight. Place the left hand in front of the right, palms facing forward at shoulder level, in front of the chest. The right palm touches the back of the left hand. In a monotone, chant the mantra:
HAR GUROO SIREE GUROO WHAA-HAY GUROO for **1 minute**.

10. In the same posture, using the same chant, lean forward from the waist. Bend a third of the way down as *HAR GUROO* is chanted. On *SIREE GUROO*, come two-thirds the way down. On *WHAA-HAY GUROO* touch the hands and head to the ground (maintaining the mudra.) Come up very quickly, and continue without breaking the rhythm. **5-6 minutes**.

11. In the same posture, with the arms touching the ground, begin a heavy Breath of Fire for **1 minute**. Then relax the breath and rest in this posture for **1-3 minutes**, as you say your own silent prayer.

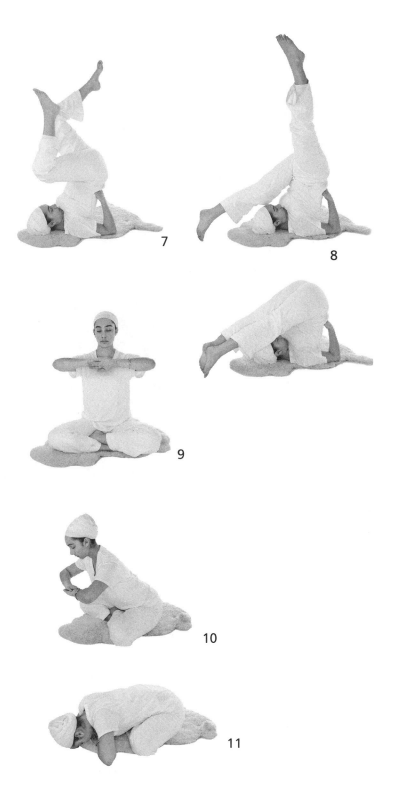

About This Kriya

When the lymph glands aren't doing their job, and the lungs aren't working properly, dead cells and mucous in the lungs, do not clear out. If this continues, ultimately you could get seriously ill. In ancient scripture there was a saying: "When anything above the Navel Point goes wrong, it is almost always a permanent problem. Below the Navel Point, a problem can always be cured."

SELF-ADJUSTMENT OF THE SPINE

AUGUST 1977

1. **Tree Pose**. Come into a standing position with the palms together at the Heart Center (Prayer Pose). Raise the left leg and place the foot on the right thigh so the heel touches the groin. **2 minutes**.

Bring the palms together over the head. Totally stretch the arms up keeping the elbows straight. **2 minutes**.

Switch legs and repeat the sequence for **2 minutes** each.

Ideally, the heel of the raised foot is resting on the pubic bone. The body is balanced with the spine firm. There will be a pressure at the base of the spine and all the vertabrae will automatically be adjusted. Women, more than men, have this capacity to adjust themselves. This exercise is also good for women's menstrual problems.

2. Stand straight with the heels together and toes pointing out at 60 degrees from the midline of the body. Interlace the fingers and place the palms on top of the head. Bend the knees and lower the torso all the way down, keeping the heels on the ground. The buttocks will be about 2-3 inches above the ground. The spine will be kept straight, though the lower back will bend forward slightly for balance. The eyes look straight ahead for balance. Inhale down and exhale up.

Rhythm: 5 seconds down, 5 seconds up per cycle. **21 complete cycles.**

The angle of the back in this exercise will allow the discs of the lower spine to adjust and balance themselves.

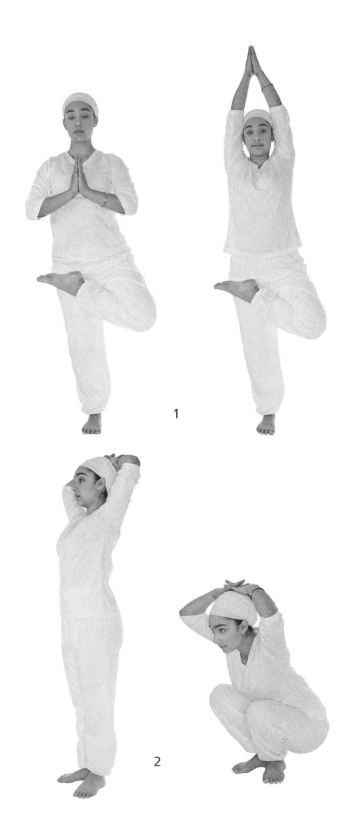

1

2

3. In a standing position, spread the legs wide apart. Bend forward from the waist and grab the toes with the hands. Let the knees bend outside of the arms and bring the back parallel to the ground, keeping the head up. Bounce the lower back and hips up and down 11 times, inhaling up, exhaling down. The position of the head does not change. Stand up and breathe normally for 5 seconds, and resume bouncing another 11 times.

Rhythm: **11 bounces per 7-8 seconds.**
TIME: 3 minutes.

This exercise corrects the sciatic nerve in the thighs, and there is no other system which can make this correction as well as this simple exercise can. Normally the sciatic nerve should never hurt in a woman, and it only hurts if it is out of place. This exercise will help to lessen the pain of the sciatic nerve in woman during cramps, menstruation, intercourse, and any other activity which affects this nerve.

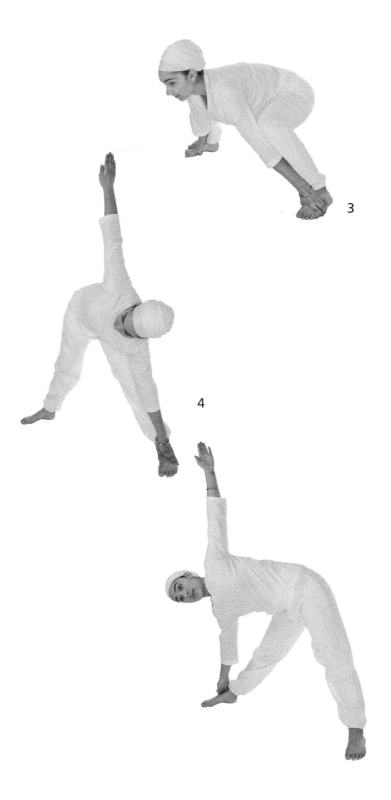

4. Stand up straight and spread the legs apart as far as possible. Totally stretch sideways to the right bringing the left arm up and over the head. Do not let it bend. The right arm stretches down towards the right foot. Switch sides and stretch to the left.

Rhythm: Hold the stretched position **10 seconds** each time, switching sides slowly without stopping in between.
TIME: 2-3 minutes.

This exercise is very helpful in correcting the balance of the musculoskeletal systems of the neck.

ADJUST YOUR FLOW
THE FOUR U's FOR YOU

JULY 5, 1984

1. Lie down flat on the back. Raise the legs and arms straight up to 90 degrees. Point the toes. Knees and elbows are straight. **11 minutes**.

Hold steady and think about what good you have done since you have come to the planet Earth. Reconcile activities with your beautiful intelligence. We are moving the life force energy today and without any movement. Keep yourself in the posture, no matter what. The energy will adjust itself.

2. Still lying on the back, bring the hands straight up over the head on the ground. Then raise the lower body up into a modified Plow Pose, with the legs straight over the head but parallel to the ground. **11 minutes**.

This is a simple flow of energy, a simple way of just being.

3. Come sitting up and stretch the legs out in front, the arms extend toward the toes, palms down and parallel to the ground. The back is straight and steady, like a statue. **11 minutes**.

The pain and disturbance comes in the adjustment of the pranic energy. You feel the pressure of the muscles adjusting themselves. Chinese call it "chi" energy, Japanese call it "qi" energy, and we call it "ji" energy. "Ji" means the soul, the inner Self, the being. Meditate, chant and recite anything mentally or verbally, but keep the posture perfect.

4. Stand up straight and bend over at the waist so the torso is parallel to the ground. Keep the back and neck straight. The arms will hang loosely down towards the ground. Form a "U" with your body. Don't bend down to the toes. You can chant or meditate to keep yourself going. **11 minutes.**

5. **Deep Relaxation**. Relax flat on the back. Listen to a gong, if available. **10 minutes**.

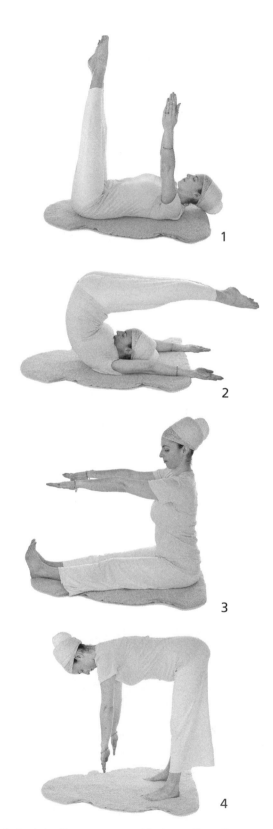

About This Kriya

This is the set of U. It invigorates you by adjusting your Pranic Body with your Auric Body in direct contrast with the Arcline. These are called the 4 U's and they are *"for you."* Anytime you do these, you need to do a deep relaxation afterwards.

Resources

Music, Manuals & More

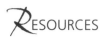

More About "I Am a Woman"

I Am A Woman: Creative, Sacred & Invincible
Selections from Yogi Bhajan appear alongside the stories and shared experiences of women from all different walks of life who have come into relationship with their True Self and these teachings.

I Am a Woman: Practicing Kindness
A DVD Series based on lectures from the Khalsa Women's Training Camp years. Practicing Kindness focuses on how kindness manifests in a woman's life: career, family, and within herself.

Volume 1: *Create Your Reality*
From June 25, 2001, includes the meditation: The Radiant Body—The Beauty of Every Woman
Volume 2: *Spiritual Acceleration*
From July 3, 2000, includes the meditation: Power Your Life Force
Volume 3: *Act Great and Never Be Turned by Fate*
From June 30, 1997, includes the meditation: Interconnected Mental Trance
Volume 4: *Know Yourself*
From July 25, 1989, includes the meditation: Receiving the Virtues
Volume 5: *The Art of Appreciation*
A rare, early video from June 27, 1984

I Am a Woman and the Khalsa Women's Training Camp Notes Online Resource
In addition to these great products for women, the Kundalini Research Institute in partnership with The Yogi Bhajan Library of Teachings, will release the complete set of KWTC notes by the end of 2009.

Music: The Classics

Meditations for the Aquarian Age by Nirinjan Kaur: an essential collection for any Kundalini Yoga Practitioner, includes Aquarian March for the Meditation for an Invincible Spirit in Chapter Four. Other classics from Nirinjan Kaur include: *Humee Hum Brahm Hum* and *Ong Namo Guru Dev Namo.*
Tantric Har by Simran Kaur Khalsa is another essential tool for any Kundalini Yogi's collection.
Rakhe Rakhanhaar by Singh Kaur. This version was Yogi Bhajan's favorite; he was instrumental in its production and sound current. There are several other beautiful versions which can be found on any Aquarian Sadhana album.
Ajai Alai by Gurushabad Singh. Newer versions by SatKirn Kaur and Mata Mandir Singh have naad that is also in alignment with the *Naad* of the original *bani.*
Promises and *Himalaya* by Sat Peter Singh
Narayan Shabd by Guru Raj Kaur
Nobel Woman by Raghu Rai Kaur; a new release of this song by SatKirn Kaur is available on *Blessings of a Woman.*
Bangara Rhythms or *Punjabi Drums* were also classics that Yogi Bhajan used in many of his classes.

Other Music & Mantra

Adi Shakti: There are many versions—choose your favorite with a classic 8-count, driving beat for best results when meditating or using during a kriya.

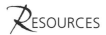

Triple Mantra is available from Gurunam Singh Levy

33rd Pauri: Snatam Kaur's *Shanti*, Sat Kirn's *Universal Prayer*

Jap Man Sat Nam: Dev Suroop Kaur's *Kundalini Beat* or Snatam Kaur's *Anand*

Sat Kartar Kaur has a version of *Jap Man Sat Nam* on her album *Listen*. She also has other beautiful 3HO music for all kinds of kriyas and meditations. *Har Har Amritsar* is a lovely meditation on the Golden Temple.

Sopurkh: Nirinjan Kaur's *Sopurkh*, 11 recitations & English translation; also a lyrical version available by Sangeet Kaur Khalsa

Bowing *Jaap Sahib*: SatKirn Kaur's *Jaap*, Sangeet Kaur and Sat Nirmal Kaur's *Jaap Sahib*, and the classic that Yogi Bhajan often played in class was by Ragi Sat Nam Singh

Ra Ma Da Sa: SatKirn Kaur's *Universal Mantra*, Snatam also has a beautiful version

Healing the Wounds of Love: Guru Raj Kaur's *Healing the Wounds of Love*; Sat Purkh's *Nectar of the Name*

Dhan Dhan Ram Das Gur: Again, there are so many beautiful versions available. Sangeet Kaur's is the classic; but find any version you like and meditate.

Bhand Jamee-ai is available on SatKirn Kaur's *Blessings of a Woman*.

Japji: Song of the Soul by Guru Raj Kaur. A beautiful 2-CD recording with musical version, English version, 3 recitations

Japji: Mata Mandir Singh also has a beautiful version in both Gurmukhi and English.

As this is being written, Snatam Kaur has a forthcoming album that focus on mantras for women. Check it out.

The Kundalini Research Institute has a pronunciation guide on its website: www.kundaliniresearchinstitute.org. Look for Tools for Teachers and Students. *Mantras of the Master* is also available from Santokh Singh; and forthcoming mantra pronunciation guide from Guru Dass Kaur will be available soon as well.

Books, Yoga Manuals & More

Japji: The Song of the Soul and *Anand Sahib* are both available in translation by Ek Ong Kaar Kaur Khalsa.

Kundalini Yoga Sadhana Guidelines, 2nd Edition, by the Kundalini Research Institute

Praana, Praanee, Praanayam edited by Harijot Kaur Khalsa

More Yoga manuals by Harijot Kaur: *Infinity & Me, Physical Wisdom, Reaching Me in Me, Self-Experience, Self-Knowledge*, and *Owner's Manual*

Kundalini Yoga: The Flow of Eternal Power by Shakti Parwha Kaur Khalsa

Excel & Celebrate by Pritpal Kaur Khalsa

Lunar Woman by Hari Charn Kaur Khalsa

Lunar Woman (DVD) by Shakta Kaur

The Art of Making Sex Sacred by Jiwan Joti Kaur Khalsa, PhD

Marriage on the Spiritual Path by Shakti Parwha Kaur Khalsa

Breathwalk® by Gurucharan Singh Khalsa, PhD and Yogi Bhajan, PhD

Conscious Pregnancy by Tarn Taran Kaur Khalsa

WomanHeart and retreats by Sangeet Kaur Khalsa

Dying into Life: The Yoga of Death, Loss and Transformation by Guru Terath Kaur Khalsa, PhD (aka Jiwan Joti Kaur Khalsa, PhD)

Other Resources

If you don't find a specific reference to a recommended version of a mantra or shabd, please see www.sikhdharma.org or www.sikhnet.com. Here you'll find a vast resource of mantras, *shabds*, and *banis* that you can download or listen to online.

Your first source for Kundalini Yoga books, manuals, and DVDs is The Kundalini Research Institute—your Source for Kundalini Yoga as taught by Yogi Bhajan®. See www.kundaliniresearchinstitute.org.

Great sources for music are www.spiritvoyage.com and www.a-healing.com.

Senior Editorial Board

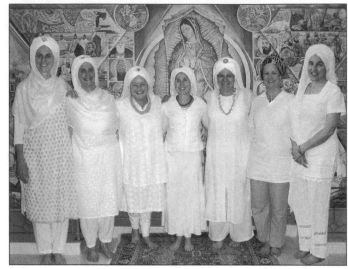

Dev Suroop Kaur Khalsa delights in the pure practicality of applying the teachings of Yogi Bhajan to create a successful, authentic, and spiritual life. An accomplished musician, recording artist, and a Professional Level Trainer in the KRI Aquarian Trainer Academy, Dev Suroop Kaur strives to break it down, keep it real, and guide students to their own empowered authenticity. From the deeply contemplative compositions in her recording, *Narayan*, to the hip, edgy beats of her chant-rap album *Kundalini Beat*, Dev Suroop Kaur offers an extraordinary range of styles to invoke the experience of the Divine Spirit. She currently lives with her husband of 25 years in Española, New Mexico and, in addition to her teaching and music activities, works to maintain a peaceful mind as a business executive. Dev Suroop Kaur is an ordained Minister of Sikh Dharma, is certified as a Registered Yoga Teacher (RYT) through Yoga Alliance, and holds a Masters of Business Administration from the Claremont Graduate University.

Deva Kaur Khalsa is a Lead Trainer in the KRI Aquarian Trainer Academy, a member of the Kundalini Research Institute's Teacher Training Executive Committee, and a member of KRI's Board of Directors. She has served the Kundalini Yoga community in Miami and Ft. Lauderdale, Florida, for more than 35 years. Joining the ashram when she was just 17, she has served the women's teachings and teacher training tirelessly over the years. With her husband Deva Singh Khalsa, she has two beautiful children, both graduates of Miri Piri Academy and currently living in Eugene, Oregon. She is co-owner of Yoga Source in Coral Springs, Florida and can be reached through www.MyYogaSource.com.

Guru Raj Kaur Khalsa was one of Yogi Bhajan's early students, and has been dedicated to perpetuating the Teachings of Kundalini Yoga and Sikh Dharma, and community building for almost 40 years. She is a Lead Trainer in the KRI Aquarian Trainer Academy and a member of the Kundalini Research Institute's Teacher Training Executive Committee; she teaches internationally along with an annual Level One Teacher Training in Vancouver, B.C. She is Founder and Director of 3HO Vancouver, Yoga West Vancouver, and Camp Raj Yog, the Sacred Land development near Vancouver. She lovingly directs Khalsa Ladies Camp, Vancouver —now in its 18th year—and the inspiring Khalsa Ladies' Camp India Yatras for women. She serves on the Sikh Dharma International Board, and bows in service as a Sikh Dharma Minister, and through the singing of Gurbani Kirtan. By profession, she is a graphic artist. She is married to Hari Singh Khalsa, and the mother of two awesome daughters: Ong Kar Kaur and Nirinjan Kaur. To find out about outstanding Vancouver programs go to: yogawest.ca, khalsaladiescamp.com, khalsamen.com, camprajyog.com.

Hari Charan Kaur Khalsa currently serves as the Kundalini Research Institute's Director of Reach Out–Teach Out programs. She is a member of the management team at Kundalini Research Institute, as well as the Kundalini Research Institute's Teacher Training Executive Committee and a Lead Trainer in Aquarian Teacher Training program. Author of *Lunar Woman*, she was blessed to attend Khalsa Women's Training Camp in Española for many years and study the women's teachings directly with Yogi Bhajan. She has traveled extensively in the international community, meeting and greeting women from all continents, and she has served the community of 3HO women for more than 35 years. Her passion remains in serving and supporting the next generation of women—and the women's teachings.

Pritpal Kaur Khalsa is a Lead Trainer in the Aquarian Teacher Training Program and a specialist in posture and alignment instruction. Author of *Excel & Celebrate: A Sacred Circle of Women*, she facilitates and coaches women's groups around the world through the technology of Kundalini Yoga as taught by Yogi Bhajan®. She currently serves as Lead Trainer in several Level 1 and Level 2 Teacher Training Programs from North Carolina to Brazil. She serves on the 3HO International Women's Camp planning committee and has served the teachings of Yogi Bhajan for more than 30 years. She has two beautiful children with her husband Pritpal Singh Khalsa, a musician, Life Coach and fellow Teacher Trainer.

Tarn Taran Kaur Khalsa is a Lead Trainer in the KRI Aquarian Trainer Academy; she and her husband travel and teach internationally throughout the year. For many years, she served as the Director of 3HO women and continues to serve the international community of women through her Conscious Pregnancy Teacher Training specialty courses. Author of *Conscious Pregnancy*, her groundbreaking work in the field of pre- and post-natal yoga continues to serve and uplift generations of women, mothers and their children. A mother, and grandmother herself, her daughter, Madhur Nain is also a KRI Certified Kundalini Yoga Teacher and an Associate Trainer in the KRI Aquarian Trainer Academy. For more information see: www.kundaliniwomen.org.

Contributors

Ek Ong Kaar Kaur Khalsa is a teacher and a writer. With a degree in Asian Studies from Rice University, Ek Ong Kaar brings her deep love of spirituality and language to the task of translating the Siri Guru Granth Sahib into English. Ek Ong Kaar served on Yogi Bhajan's staff for several years prior to his passing in 2004. During that time Yogi Bhajan guided her in how to approach translating the writings of the Sikh Masters. As a Sikh Dharma Minister and Creative Director for Sikh Dharma International, Ek Ong Kaar travels and teachers regularly. Author of contemporary and scholarly translations of *Japji Sahib: The Song of the Soul* and *Anand Sahib: The Song of Bliss*, her work reaches into the heart and soul of the reader and brings you to the feet of your own inner wisdom.

Sat Purkh Kaur Khalsa is a writer, editor, poet, singer and songwriter—and a pretty good cook, too. She is a KRI Certified Kundalini Yoga Level One Teacher and an Associate Trainer in the KRI Aquarian Trainer Academy, specializing in Naad. Sat Purkh joined the KRI staff in 2006 and was instrumental in the development of the Level Two Teacher Training curriculums. Currently she serves the Yogi Bhajan Library of Teachings Capital Campaign as well as Editor and Product Development Director for KRI and recently served on the 3HO International Women's Camp planning committee. Her album, *Nectar of the Name*, was released in 2007 and her new single, *Jai Ma!*, is available at www.kundaliniresearchinstitute.org. She lives with her two cats, Fatty and Slim, and her dog Vinnie.

A Brief Guide to Commonly Used
YOGA TERMS

As you approach the remarkable sets and meditations in this Manual, you will notice some frequently used terms. If you are a Kundalini Yogi, you may be familiar with these terms. If you haven't yet studied Kundalini Yoga as taught by Yogi Bhajan®, here is a brief introduction to terms. For best results in your practice, we encourage everyone to study with a KRI certified Kundalini Yoga teacher in your local community.

Amrit Vela: Literally "ambrosial time." The 2-1/2 hours before the rising of the sun. During this special time you are most receptive to the soul; you can clear the subconscious of wrong habits and impulses; and you can connect with the teachers and saints from all traditions. It is the best time to perform sadhana (spiritual discipline).

Arcline: One of 10 bodies of a human being. It is a thin bright arc, like a halo, that goes from ear to ear over the forehead near the normal hairline. It reflects the interaction of the soul of the person with its vital energy resources, and in it are written the potential, destiny, and health of the person. Women have a second Arcline from nipple to nipple. See page 20 and 114 for more information.

Aura: One of the 10 bodies, the Aura is the radiant field of energy and consciousness that surrounds the physical body and which holds and organizes the seven centers of energy called chakras. Its strength, measured by brightness and radius, determines the vitality and integrity of a person.

Bana: Clothing which projects a particular consciousness.

Breath of Fire: One of the foundational breath techniques used in the practice of Kundalini Yoga. It accompanies many postures, and has numerous beneficial effects. It is important to master this breath so that it is done accurately and becomes automatic. See page 152 for detailed instructions.

Chakra: The word connotes a wheel in action. It usually refers to the seven primary energy centers in the aura that align along the spine from the base to the top of the skull. Each chakra is a center of consciousness with a set of values, concerns, and powers of action associated with it.

Easy Pose: This is a simple but stable yogic sitting posture. It is sitting cross-legged "tailor fashion," but with a yogic awareness of keeping the spine straight, with the lower spine slightly forward so the upper spine can stay straight.

Gyan Mudra: The most commonly used mudra for meditation. The tip of the thumb touches the tip of the Jupiter (index) finger. This stimulates knowledge, wisdom, and the power to compute. The energy of the index finger is associated with Jupiter, representing expansion. Its qualities are receptivity and calm.

Golden Chain of Teachers or the Golden Link: Historically it is the long line of spiritual masters who have preceded us. Practically it is the subtle link between the consciousness of a student and the master, which has the power to guide and protect the energy of a teaching and its techniques. This link requires the student to put aside the ego and limitations and act in complete synchrony or devotion to the highest consciousness of the master and the teachings.

Ida: One of the three major channels (nadis) for subtle energy in the body. It is associated with the flow of breath through the left nostril and represents the qualities of the moon—calmness, receptivity, coolness, and imagination. It is associated with the functions of the parasympathetic nervous system but is not identical to it nor derived from it.

Jalandar Bandh also called Neck Lock: This is the most basic of the locks. It is a general rule to apply it in all chanting meditations and during most pranayams. Whenever you are holding the breath in or out, it is usually applied unless instructed otherwise. Sit comfortably with the spine straight. Lift the chest and sternum upward. Gently stretch the back of the neck straight by pulling the chin toward the back of the neck. The head stays level and centered, and does not tilt forward or to either side. The muscles of the neck and throat remain loose. Keep the muscles of the face and brow relaxed.

Japji Sahib: An inspired poem, or scripture composed by Guru Nanak. *Japji Sahib* provides a view of the cosmos, the soul, the mind, the challenge of life, and describes the impact of our actions. Its 40 stanzas are thea source of many mantras and can be used as a whole or in part to guide both your mind and your heart.

Japa: Literally "to repeat." It is the conscious, alert, and precise repetition of a mantra.

Kriya: Literally means "completed action." An integrated sequence of postures, breath, and sound that work together to manifest a particular state. Kundalini Yoga as taught by Yogi Bhajan® is structured in kriyas, a sequence of postures and yoga techniques used to produce a particular impact on the psyche, body, or self. The structure of each kriya has been designed to generate, organize, and deliver a particular state or change of state, thereby completing a cycle of effect.

Kundalini Yoga: A Raj Yoga that creates vitality in the body, balance in the mind, and openness to the spirit. It is used by the house-holder, busy in the world, to create immediate clarity. The fourth Guru in the Sikh tradition, Guru Ram Das, was acknowledged as the greatest Raj Yogi. He opened this long-secret tradition to all.

Long Deep Breathing: One of the most basic yogic breaths. It uses the full capacity of the lungs. Long Deep Breathing starts by filling the abdomen, then expanding the chest, and finally lifting the upper ribs and clavicle. The exhale is the reverse: first the upper deflates, then the middle, and finally the abdomen pulls in and up, as the Navel Point pulls back toward the spine.

Mantra: Sounds or words that tune or control the mind. Man means mind. Trang is the wave or movement of the mind. Mantra is a wave, a repetition of sound and rhythm that directs or controls the mind. When you recite a mantra you have impact: through the meridian points in the mouth, through its meaning, through its pattern of energy, through its rhythm, and through its naad—energetic shape in time. Recited correctly a mantra will activate areas of the nervous system and brain and allow you to shift your state and the perceptual vision or energetic ability associated with it.

Mudra: Mudra means "seal." It usually refers to hand positions used in meditation and exercise practices. These hand positions are used to seal the body's energy flow in a particular pattern. More generally it can refer to other locks, bandhas and meditation practices that seal the flow of energy.

Mulbandh: This literally means "root lock" and Root Lock is commonly used to refer to mulbandh and is routinely used in Kundalini Yoga. It is a body lock used to balance prana and apana at the Navel Point. This releases reserve energy which is used to arouse the kundalini. It is a contraction of the lower pelvis—the navel point, the sex organs, and the rectum. It coordinates, stimulates, and balances the energies in the lower triangle (first three chakras). This bandh is frequently applied at the end of an exercise or kriya to crystallize its effects. Root Lock is a smooth motion that consists of three parts: First contract the anal sphincter. Feel the muscles lift upward and inward. Once these muscles tighten and move, contract the area around the sex organ. This is experienced as a slight lift and inward rotation of the pubic bone, similar to stopping the flow of urine or Kegel exercises. Then contract the lower abdominal muscles and the Navel Point toward the spine. These three actions are applied together in a smooth, rapid, flowing, motion.

Naad: The inner sound that is subtle and all-present. It is the direct expression of the Absolute. Meditated upon, it pulls the consciousness toward expansion.

Naam: The manifested identity of the essence. The word derives from *Naa-ay-ma*, which means "that which is not, now is born." A Naam gives identity, form, and expression to that which was only essence. It is also referred to as the Word.

Nadi: Channels or pathways of subtle energy. It is said that there are over 72,000 primary nadis throughout the body.

Navel Point: The sensitive area of the body just below the umbilicus that accumulates and stores life force energy, also known in Eastern martial art traditions as the hara. It is the reserve energy from this area that initiates the flow of the kundalini energy from the base of the spine. If the navel area is strong, your vital force and health are also strong.

Negative Mind: One of the three Functional Minds. It is the fastest and acts to defend you. It asks, "How can this harm me? How can this limit or stop me?" It is also the power to just say no, stop something, or reject a direction of action.

Neutral Mind: The most refined and often the least developed of the three Functional Minds. It judges and assesses. It witnesses and gives you clarity. It holds the power of intuition and the ability to see your purpose and destiny. It is the gateway for awareness.

Panj Shabd: Panj means five: Sa Ta Na Ma, that is S, T, N, M, A. It is the "atomic" or naad form of the mantra Sat Nam. It is used to increase intuition, balance the hemispheres of the brain, and to create a destiny for someone when there was none.

Pavan Guru: Literally, the "breath of the guru." It is the transformative wisdom that is embedded in the patterns of breath, especially those patterns generated in the expression of naad, in sound or mantra.

Pingala: One of the three major channels (nadis) for subtle energy in the body. It is associated with the flow of breath through the right nostril and represents the qualities of the sun—energy, heat, action, and projective power. It is associated with the functions of the sympathetic nervous system but is not identical to it or derived from it.

Positive Mind: One of the three Functional Minds. It elaborates, magnifies, extends, and assists. It asks, "How can this help me? How can I use this? What is the positive side of this?"

Prana: The universal life force that gives motion. It is the breath in air. It is the subtle breath of the purusha as it vibrates with a psycho-physical energy or presence. Prana regulates the modes and moods of the mind.

Pranayam: Regulated breathing patterns or exercises.

Pratyahar: One of the eight limbs of yoga, it is the synchronization of the thoughts with the Infinite. To quote Yogi Bhajan: "*Pratyahar* is the control of the mind through the withdrawal of the senses. The joy in your life, which you really want to enjoy, is within you. There is nothing more precise than you within you. The day you find the you within you, your mind will be yours. In *pratyahar* we bring everything to zero (*shuniya*), as pranayam brings everything to Infinity."

Sadhana: A spiritual discipline; the early morning practice of yoga, meditation, and other spiritual exercises.

Sat: Existence; what is; the subtle essence of Infinity itself; often translated as Truth.

Sat Nam: The essence or seed embodied in form; the identity of truth. When used as a greeting it means "I greet and salute that reality and truth which is your soul." It is called the Bij Mantra—the seed for all that comes.

Shabd: Sound, especially subtle sound or sound imbued with consciousness. It is a property or emanation of consciousness itself. If you meditate on shabd it awakens your awareness.

Shabd Guru: These are sounds spoken by the Gurus; the vibration of the Infinite Being which transforms your consciousness; the sounds and words captured by the Gurus in the writings which comprise the Siri Guru Granth Sahib.

Shakti: The creative power and principle of existence itself. Without it nothing can manifest or bloom. It is feminine in nature.

Shuniya: A state of the mind and consciousness where the ego is brought to zero or complete stillness. There a power exists. It is the fundamental power of a Kundalini Yoga teacher. When you become shuniya then the One will carry you. You do not grasp or act. With folded hands you "are not." It is then that Nature acts for you.

Sushmana: One of the three major channels (nadis) for subtle energy in the body. It is associated with the central channel of the spine and is the place of neutrality through which the Kundalini travels when awakened. When mantra is vibrated from this place it has the power of soul and consciousness.

Sikh Gurus: In the Sikh tradition there were 10 living Gurus and one Guru, the Shabd Guru—the Word that guided and flowed through each of them. This succession of 10 Gurus revealed the Sikh path over a 200-year period. They were:

1st Sikh Guru: Guru Nanak	6th Sikh Guru: Guru Hargobind
2nd Sikh Guru: Guru Angad	7th Sikh Guru: Guru Har Rai
3rd Sikh Guru: Guru Amar Das	8th Sikh Guru: Guru Har Krishan
4th Sikh Guru: Guru Ram Das	9th Sikh Guru: Guru Teg Bahadur
5th Sikh Guru: Guru Arjan	10th Sikh Guru: Guru Gobind Singh

The 10th Sikh Guru, Guru Gobind Singh, passed the Guruship to the Siri Guru Granth Sahib, which embodies the writings, teachings, and sound current of the Gurus.

Simran: A deep meditative process in which the naam of the Infinite is remembered and dwelled in without conscious effort.

Siri Guru Granth Sahib: Sacred compilation of the words of the Sikh Gurus as well as of Hindu, Muslim, Sufi, and other saints. It captures the expression of consciousness and truth derived when in a state of divine union with God. It is written in naad and embodies the transformative power and structure of consciousness in its most spiritual and powerful clarity. It is a source of many mantras.

Tattvas: A category of cosmic existence; a stage of reality or being; a "thatness" of differentiated qualities. In total there are 36 tattvas. Each wave of differentiation has its own rules and structure. The final five tattvas are called the gross elements and have the phasic qualities and relationships of ether, air, fire, water, and earth.

Ten Bodies: We are all spiritual beings having a human experience. In order to have this experience the spirit takes on 10 bodies or vehicles. They are the Soul Body, the three Mental Bodies (Negative, Positive, and Neutral Minds), the Physical Body, Pranic Body, Arcline Body, Auric Body, Subtle Body, and Radiant Body. Each body has its own quality, function, and realm of action.

Third Eye Point: The sixth chakra or center of consciousness. It is located at a point on the forehead between the eyebrows. Associated with the functioning of the pituitary gland, it is the command center and integrates the parts of the personality. It gives you insight, intuition, and the understanding of meanings and impacts beyond the surface of things. For this reason it is the focal point in many meditations.

Uddiyana bandh or Diaphragm Lock: The name of this lock comes from a Sanskrit word which means "to fly up." In this bandh, the energy of the lower abdomen rises. The uddiyana bandh crosses the mind-body barrier, vertically integrating the emotional qualities and allowing circulation of the pranic energy into the central channel, the *sushmuna*. Diaphragm Lock is only applied on the exhale. Pull the entire abdominal region, especially the area above the Navel Point, upward and back towards the spine.

Wahe Guru: A mantra of ecstasy and dwelling in God. It is the Infinite teacher of the soul. Also called the Gur Mantra.

Yogi: One who has attained a state of yoga (union) where polarities are mastered and transcended. One who practices the disciplines of yoga and has attained self-mastery.